SAGE was founded in 1965 by Sara Miller McCune to support the dissemination of usable knowledge by publishing innovative and high-quality research and teaching content. Today, we publish over 900 journals, including those of more than 400 learned societies, more than 800 new books per year, and a growing range of library products including archives, data, case studies, reports, and video. SAGE remains majority-owned by our founder, and after Sara's lifetime will become owned by a charitable trust that secures our continued independence.

Los Angeles | London | New Delhi | Singapore | Washington DC | Melbourne

Advance Praise

Home-grown vaccines have helped India overcome the mammoth, unprecedented challenge posed by the COVID-19 pandemic. Domestic R&D and manufacturing have produced vaccines which have effectively blunted the sting of many other infectious diseases too. In this book, Dr Yadav has not only presented several fascinating stories behind the development of vaccines but also provided the readers a spread of diverse and topical issues surrounding vaccines. It's a comprehensive and valuable treatise which should find a place in every bookshelf.

—Rajesh Bhushan
Secretary, Ministry of Health & Family Welfare
Government of India

Dr Sajjan Yadav's book is an illuminating account of the growth journey of vaccines spanning over two centuries. Vaccines are among the most profound public health tools to reduce and eradicate infectious diseases. The ravaging COVID-19 pandemic has highlighted the power of vaccines in saving lives and yet, quite ironically, anti-vaccine sentiment is becoming a growing threat. Dr Yadav eloquently conveys the value of vaccine equity, both between and within countries, and digs deep into India's impressive achievement in developing, producing and distributing COVID-19 vaccines. It is a highly recommended read for everyone interested in a one-stop read on vaccines.

—Anuradha Gupta
Deputy CEO
Gavi, the Vaccine Alliance

Vaccines, undoubtedly, are the key to global health security and sustainable development. Equitable access to effective and safe vaccines is vital not only to end the ongoing COVID-19 pandemic but also to save millions of lives annually. In this deeply researched book, Dr Sajjan Yadav presents the stories of development of vaccines from scratch and narrates with ease the tale of transformation of India into a vaccine superpower. His bird's eye view on the subject put out in a simple and interesting language presents a captivating account of the development of vaccines for COVID-19 at a pandemic speed and conduct of the world's largest vaccination drive by India. This page turner also delves upon many novel concepts such as vaccine diplomacy, vaccine economy, vaccine equity, vaccine nationalism and vaccine leadership. The book will be of immense interest to a wide variety of audience, including health professionals, students, administrators and the audience looking to understand the subject in detail.

—Professor Randeep Guleria

Director, All India Institute of Medical Sciences,
New Delhi

This book packs in a delightful tale on vaccines with nuggets of important information associated with them. This brilliant compilation not just tells the birthing stories of various vaccines but also delves upon the whole gamut of issues surrounding the topic starting from their social and economic benefits to the impact of 'Vaccine Maitri' on international relations. I'd highly recommend it for all readers interested to know the history and science behind this lifesaver.

—Professor (Dr) Balram Bhargava

Secretary, Department of Health Research
Director General, Indian Council of Medical Research

Immunization is a cornerstone of public health policy. In *India's Vaccine Growth Story*, Dr Yadav has given us a highly readable account of the colourful history of vaccines and vaccination, which is both educational and entertaining: From cowpox to

COVID-19, this book is a must-have for anyone seeking a better understanding of viruses and immunology. It will certainly make a valuable addition to every growing family's home library.

—Dr Phil Edwards
Associate Professor of Epidemiology & Statistics,
London School of Hygiene & Tropical Medicine

Arriving at the right time, this book tells the birthing stories of various vaccines and their benefits to mankind and also explains the vaccine leadership, vaccine nationalism, hesitancy, eagerness and equity. It is a must-read and must-have for policymakers, medical practitioners, researchers, public health officials and, of course, every concerned citizen who should know that how science has been saving millions of people every year from infectious demons starting from smallpox to COVID-19.

—Shyamlal Yadav
Senior Editor, The Indian Express

Sajjan Singh Yadav has presented the vaccine story in an uncomplicated way, alongside the history and geography of vaccine production, worldwide. Coupled with stories of national prowess and humanitarian outreach, the book is a useful compendium for those involved in the formulation and execution of vaccine programmes or pursuing education and research. The author's civil service background has enabled him to think laterally, although a penchant for India's achievements is discernible.

—Shailaja Chandra
Former Secretary in the Ministry of Health,
Government of India
Former Chief Secretary, Delhi

The last few decades have shown us that efficacious, safe and cost-effective vaccines are a powerful tool to overcome many global health challenges, including eradicating disease. India's emergence as a vaccine superpower has greatly contributed to the widespread global availability of affordable, high-quality vaccines which help save countless lives across the world. In this well-researched and comprehensive volume on India's vaccines story, Dr Yadav weaves a compelling narrative about this journey and future opportunities. This book is an essential reading for anyone interested in public health and the role of Indian innovation.

—Hari Menon
Country Director–India, Bill & Melinda Gates Foundation

INDIA'S VACCINE GROWTH STORY

INDIA'S VACCINE GROWTH STORY

From Cowpox to Vaccine Maitri

SAJJAN SINGH YADAV

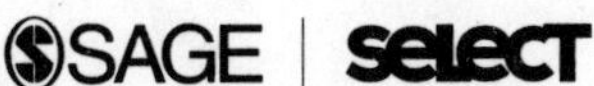

Los Angeles | London | New Delhi
Singapore | Washington DC | Melbourne

First published in 2022 by

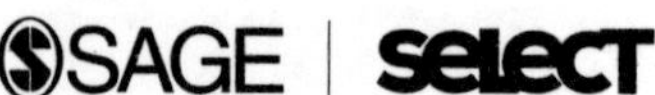

SAGE Publications India Pvt Ltd
B1/I-1 Mohan Cooperative Industrial Area
Mathura Road, New Delhi 110 044, India
www.sagepub.in

SAGE Publications Inc
2455 Teller Road
Thousand Oaks, California 91320, USA

SAGE Publications Ltd
1 Oliver's Yard, 55 City Road
London EC1Y 1SP, United Kingdom

SAGE Publications Asia-Pacific Pte Ltd
18 Cross Street #10-10/11/12
China Square Central
Singapore 048423

Published by Vivek Mehra for SAGE Publications India Pvt Ltd. Typeset in 11/14pt Adobe Caslon by Fidus Design Pvt Ltd, Chandigarh.

Library of Congress Control Number: 2022936976

ISBN: 978-93-5479-523-7 (PB)

SAGE Team: Manisha Mathews, Neena Ganjoo and Kanika Mathur

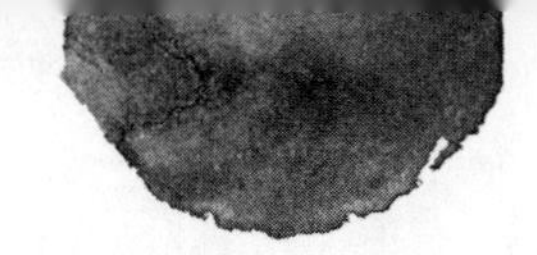

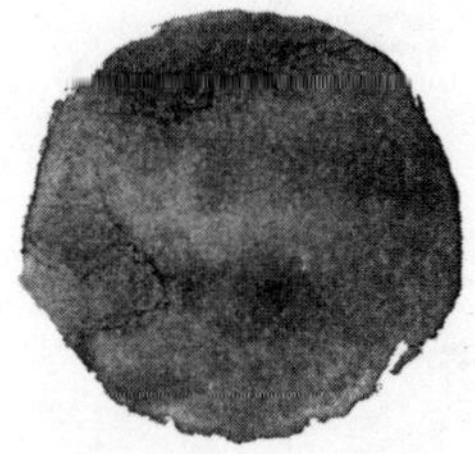

To

My lifeline, Sunita,

My darling daughter, Siya

and

My loving son, Karan.

Contents

List of Abbreviations

ACP	African, Caribbean and Pacific
ACT-A	Access to COVID-19 Tools Accelerator
AEFI	Adverse events following immunization
AIDS	Acquired immunodeficiency syndrome
AIIMS	All India Institute of Medical Sciences
AMCs	Advance market commitments
ANMs	Auxiliary nurse and midwives
APA	Advance purchase agreement
ASDs	Autism spectrum disorders
BCG	Bacillus Calmette–Guérin
BIBCOL	Bharat Immunologicals Biologicals Limited
BIRAC	Biotechnology Industry Research Assistance Council
BPL	Beta-Propiolactone
BRI	Belt and Road Initiative
BSE	Bombay Stock Exchange
CAGR	Compound annual growth rate
CARICOM	Caribbean Community
CCE	Cold chain equipment
CCP	Cold chain point
CCTs	Cold chain technicians

CDC	Centers for Disease Control and Prevention
CDLs	Central Drugs Laboratories
CDSCO	Central Drugs Standard Control Organisation
CEPI	Coalition for Epidemic Preparedness Innovations
CHAs	Community health assistants
COINEX	COVID19 Information Exchange Platform
COVAX	COVID-19 Vaccines Global Access Facility
COVID-19	Coronavirus disease 2019
CoWIN	COVID Vaccine Intelligence Network
CRI	Central Research Institute
CSIR	Council for Scientific and Industrial Research
C-TAP	COVID-19 Technology Access Pool
CVC	COVID-19 vaccination centre
DALYs	Disability-adjusted life years
DBT	Department of Biotechnology
DCGI	Drugs Controller General of India
DF	Deep freezer
DFC	Development Finance Corporation
DIKSHA	Digital Infrastructure for Knowledge Sharing
DNA	Deoxyribonucleic acid
DPT	Diphtheria, pertussis and tetanus
DOVE	Decade of Vaccine Economics
DrPH	Doctor of Public Health
EPI	Expanded Programme on Immunization
EUA	Emergency Use Authorization
eVIN	Electronic Vaccine Intelligence Network

EXIM	Export import
FDI	Foreign direct investment
FLW	Frontline worker
GAVI	Global Alliance for Vaccines and Immunization
GBS	Guillain–Barré syndrome
GCLP	Good Clinical Laboratory Practice
GDP	Gross domestic product
GMP	Good Manufacturing Practice
GPEI	Global Polio Eradication Initiative
GVAP	Global Vaccine Action Plan
HBPCL	Haffkine Biopharmaceutical Ltd
HiB	Haemophilus influenzae type B
HICs	High-income countries
HIV	Human immunodeficiency virus
HPSCI	House Permanent Select Committee on Intelligence
HPV	Human papillomavirus
ICMR	Indian Council of Medical Research
IEC	Information, Education and Communication
iGOT	Integrated Government Online Training
ILR	Ice Lined Refrigerator
IMF	International Monetary Fund
INR	Indian rupee
IPR	Intellectual property right
IPV	Inactivated polio vaccine
IT	Information technology

ITEC	Indian Technical and Economic Cooperation
ITFDE	International Task Force for Disease Eradication
IVI	International Vaccine Institute
JBIC	Japan Bank for International Cooperation
KIPM	King Institute of Preventive Medicine
LIC	Low-income country
LMIC	Lower-middle-income country
LSHTM	London School of Hygiene & Tropical Medicine
MERS	Middle East respiratory syndrome
MHRA	Medicines and Healthcare Products Regulatory Agency
MMR	Measles, mumps and rubella
MoU	Memorandum of understanding
mRNA	Messenger RNA
NCCS	National Centre for Cell Science
NEGVAC	National Expert Group on Vaccine Administration for COVID-19
NHCVCs	Near to Home COVID Vaccination Centres
NHM	National Health Mission
NIAB	National Institute of Animal Biotechnology
NIFTY	National Stock Exchange FIFTY
NMRRC	National Media Rapid Response Cell
NRA	National Regulatory Authority
NSEP	National Smallpox Eradication Program
NTDs	Neglected tropical diseases
OPV	Oral polio vaccine

OTP	One-time password
PACT	Partnerships for Accelerating Clinical Trials
PHC	Primary health centre
PLI	Production Linked Incentive
PM-CARES	Prime Minister's Citizen Assistance and Relief in Emergency Situations Fund
PPE	Personal protective equipment
PSU	Public sector undertaking
QUAD	Quadrilateral Security Dialogue
R&D	Research and development
RDIF	Russian Direct Investment Fund
RNA	Ribonucleic Acid
RWA	Resident welfare association
SAARC	South Asian Association for Regional Cooperation
SARS	Severe acute respiratory syndrome
SARS-CoV-2	Severe Acute Respiratory Syndrome Coronavirus 2
SII	Serum Institute of India
SSKs	Saheli Samanvay Kendras
TT	Tetanus toxoid
UIP	Universal Immunization Programme
UK	United Kingdom
UMIC	Upper-middle-income country
UN	United Nations
UNGA	United Nations General Assembly

UNMEER	United Nations Mission for Ebola Emergency Response
UNICEF	United Nations Children's Fund
USFDA	United States Food and Drug Administration
USP	Unique selling proposition
VEC	Vaccine Expert Committee
VPDs	Vaccine preventable diseases
WHO	World Health Organization
WIC	Walk-in cooler
WIF	Walk-in freezer
WIV	Wuhan Institute of Virology
WTO	World Trade Organization

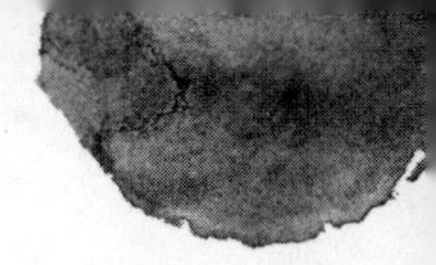

Foreword

ॐ सर्वे भवन्तु सुखिनः सर्वे सन्तु निरामयाः।

'May everybody be happy; may everybody be free from disease.'

Following this ancient 'mantra', India has been providing low-cost drugs and vaccines globally for the last four decades. The world has recognized the critical role played by our affordable medicine in the fight against many dreaded pathogens. It was not very long ago when a large number of people of low- and middle-income countries were losing life due to HIV/AIDS because they could not afford expensive drugs. At that time too, inexpensive, made-in-India medicines saved millions of lives world over.

Vaccines are the most potent weapon in the fight against infectious diseases. In recent years, humans have registered victories against many dreadful pathogens. India has successfully eliminated terrible foes such as smallpox, polio and maternal and neonatal tetanus through vaccines. These magical bullets have halted the march of numerous other microbes too.

India has a well-established capacity in development and production of vaccines. Thanks to a transformed policy environment and astounding efforts of our scientists and entrepreneurs, we are now not only 'atmanirbhar' in vaccine production but also supplying a plethora of vaccines to the entire world. It's a matter of great pride for us that every second child in the world gets the protective shield against infectious diseases through made-in-India vaccines.

Right from early 2020, the Indian government continuously engaged with Indian scientists and vaccine industry players to develop and scale up COVID-19 vaccines. Financial and technical support was provided to domestic vaccine makers through 'Mission COVID Suraksha'. Production of vaccines developed abroad was also facilitated by waiving off the requirement of bridging trials. Regulatory processes were simplified.

Our efforts bore fruit soon and we embarked upon the world's biggest vaccination drive. The drive became stronger with each passing day. The number of vaccination centres multiplied to 100,000 from 3,000. The number of people vaccinated daily touched the 8–10 million mark, more than the entire population of several countries. Breaking one record after the other, with its two home-grown vaccines, India achieved the momentous landmark of administering 1 billion jabs within 9 months. As I write this, we are moving fast towards the 2 billion mark.

In the process, we overcame tough and multifaceted challenges: vaccine hesitancy, eagerness, availability, transportation, equitable access, effective communication and expectation management, cold chain dynamics, vaccine centres logistics and so on. The drive successfully demonstrated the reach and resilience of our public health system. Experience of the universal immunization programme definitely came in handy.

I am delighted that in this book, *India's Vaccine Growth Story: From Cowpox to Vaccine Maitri*, Dr Yadav has beautifully captured the centuries-long journey of evolution of vaccines, globally. He has also elaborated the story of vaccine development in India in an interesting manner.

The book takes its readers on a fascinating roller-coaster journey of vaccines. India's story from being dependent on other countries for vaccine material to its emergence as a global vaccine superpower has been astounding. This book also educates the readers on how SARS-CoV-2 emerged, leading to development of COVID-19 vaccines at an unprecedented pace. The author has also delved upon future challenges that may emerge for vaccinology and new vistas for the growth of Indian vaccine industry in a candid manner.

Dr Yadav has a rich experience of policy formulation and implementation. This book, on a subject that is topical and of high relevance in the current times, testifies the seasoned policymaker's strong grasp on the matter.

I am sure that every reader laying hands on this book will not just enjoy it but also learn a great deal from it.

Dr Vinod K. Paul

Member, National Institute for Transforming India (NITI Aayog)

Preface

The Silver Bullet

If there's one word that defines 2021 for me and perhaps billion others across the globe, it has to be 'vaccine'. The verdict was also almost unanimous across dictionaries and search engines.[1,2,3] No one was surprised by the proclamation. It was an obvious verdict as all through the year, there was an unprecedented and mad scramble to secure vaccines for COVID-19. The jabs were the only hope to save the world from the devastating disease, which was declared a global pandemic by the World Health Organization (WHO) on 11 March 2020.[4]

THE GREATEST CATASTROPHE IN 100 YEARS

Beginning with the dawn of the year 2020, humans have fought a fierce battle for survival—one of the toughest since the emergence of *Homo sapiens* on the savannah plain about 200,000 years ago. The adversary was a new and deadly foe, the highly contagious and wicked virus named SARS-CoV-2, which caused the COVID-19 disease.[5]

Nobel Laureate and biologist Joshua Lederberg once said, 'The single biggest threat to man's continued dominance on this planet is the virus.' SARS-CoV-2, by causing the greatest economic and human devastation in history, has proved that Lederberg was right. Beginning quietly in Wuhan in the People's Republic of China towards the fag end of 2019, SARS-CoV-2 quickly made its presence felt all over the world. As early as 30 January 2020, it compelled the WHO to sound its loudest alarm: a declaration called 'public health emergency of international concern'.[6]

With no vaccine to fight the new pathogen, governments were compelled to enforce months of lockdowns. Other softer public health measures such as social distancing and adequate sanitation to control the spread of the new virus were also tried. Their success, though, was limited. Therefore, everyone pinned their hopes on potential vaccines against the scourge. The year 2020 went by, closely followed by the development of numerous vaccines.

On 2 December 2020, the world heaved a big sigh of relief when the United Kingdom's Medicines and Healthcare Products Regulatory Agency (MHRA) granted emergency use authorization to the world's first COVID-19 vaccine.[7] Many more such announcements followed. India also announced the development of two vaccines in the country. As the year 2021 unfolded, the world was ready with multiple vaccines to decimate the deadly contagion.

CONTAGIONS ARE OLD FOES OF HUMANITY

SARS-CoV-2 was not the first pathogen to challenge the existence of human beings on earth. Epidemics and pandemics have ravaged humanity since the very beginning of human civilizations. The spread of infectious diseases in the human population was accelerated by the shift from hunter–gatherers to agrarian societies.[8]

Analyses of viral DNA in ancient human remains have established that smallpox ravaged human beings for at least 3,000 years.[9] The measles virus jumped to humans in the first millennium BC.[10] We have been fighting hepatitis B and plague since the Bronze Age.[11,12] And polio has been depicted to exist in Egyptian paintings from the period 1403 to 1365 BC.[13]

Numerous contagions have claimed millions of human lives and brought suffering and misery to billions of people. At a conservative estimate, smallpox killed over 300 million people in the 20th century alone.[14] The influenza pandemic of 1918 killed 50 million people.[15] And polio paralyzed 350,000 children worldwide in 1988, when the global polio eradication drive was launched.[16]

VACCINE: ADVENT OF THE SILVER BULLET

The devastation caused by multiple pathogens would have continued unabated had we not discovered the miracle named 'vaccine'. The word 'vaccine' comes from the Latin word *vaccinus*, which means 'of or from a cow'.[17] Vaccines originated from the word *variolae vaccinae*, which means smallpox of the cow. This was because the world's first vaccine against the dreaded smallpox was made from the pus extracted from a cow pox pustule. This vaccine was discovered by English physician Edward Jenner in 1796. Jenner used the term 'vaccine' as an adjective in 1799. It was Jenner's friend Richard Dunning who coined the term 'vaccination' for the process.[18,19,20]

For the next 90 years, vaccines referred only to the inoculation of cowpox matter for smallpox.[21] In February 1880, famous French microbiologist Luis Pasteur made a presentation before the French Acade´mie des Sciences. He briefed the academy on the results of his study on protection from the virulent fowl cholera by inoculating chicken with old cultures of the causative agent. Pasteur named the phenomenon 'vaccination' in honour of Edward Jenner.[21,22]

After the discovery of the first laboratory vaccine for fowl cholera by Louis Pasteur in 1879, discoveries of vaccines picked up pace. Vaccines against rabies, cholera, plague and typhoid were available before the end of the 19th century. The 20th century witnessed the rollout of vaccines against numerous dreaded diseases. This continued with a greater vigour in the 21st century with the discovery of new platforms and the advent of new vaccine development technologies.[23]

Humans have made incredible progress in the conquest of infectious diseases. The dreaded smallpox was eliminated in 1980. Another scourge, poliomyelitis, has been tamed too and is only reported sporadically in two countries, Pakistan and Afghanistan.[24] Incidences of numerous other vaccine preventable diseases (VPDs) have also gone down substantially.

So how exactly did the silver bullet named vaccines, considered the greatest success in the history of public health, enable us to fight deadly contagions?

THE SCIENCE BEHIND VACCINES

To fight pathogens, the human body has an immune system. The system works by producing specialized proteins called antibodies by using B cells, which bind the antigen of the pathogen and neutralize it. In response to an infection, the immune system also produces T cells, which destroy the infected cells in the body. The immune system also builds a memory against the invading pathogen to immediately neutralize any reinvasion.

However, the body takes a few days to produce the right antibodies in adequate quantity to kill the pathogen. This leads to morbidity and mortality. Vaccines cut down this time lag by priming the immune system to detect and neutralize a pathogen quickly. They do this by exposing the body to a harmless version of the virus or bacteria or a part thereof (called the antigen) to recognize the hitherto unknown pathogen. The antigens induce the immune system to generate an immune response. In the event of a subsequent attack by the pathogen, the already primed immune system mounts a quick defence to block or kill it and prevents it from causing the disease. Some vaccines require multiple doses at a prescribed interval to strengthen the body's 'memory bank' to provide long-lasting protection.

Vaccines are in different genres, such as live attenuated vaccines, inactivated vaccines, subunit vaccines, recombinant vaccines and nucleic acid vaccines. Let's get acquainted with them.

LIVE ATTENUATED VACCINES

A live attenuated vaccine is produced by weakening a pathogen in a laboratory to such an extent that when administered in the body, it does not cause illness but retains its ability to grow and induce immunity. Their virulence is reduced by passing the pathogens multiple times through non-human cells.[25] Only a small dose of the pathogen is required, which replicates to produce enough organisms inside the body to stimulate an immune response. A weakened pathogen resembles a natural infection very closely and produces a strong immune response that is identical to the one produced by a natural infection.

A live attenuated vaccine is simple to design and usually needs to be administered as a single dose. However, its administration is fraught with the danger of the pathogen regaining its virulence and causing the disease, especially in the young and immune-compromised persons. Vaccines must be handled and stored carefully, since the live organisms in them are fragile and can be damaged by heat or light.[26] Examples of live attenuated vaccines include polio, measles, influenza, rubella, mumps, yellow fever, rotavirus, chicken-pox, BCG and oral typhoid vaccines.[27] The first human vaccine, the smallpox vaccine, was also a live attenuated vaccine.

INACTIVATED VACCINES: CHALLENGING IMMUNE SYSTEM WITH KILLED PATHOGENS

Inactivated vaccines are produced by growing a virus or bacterium in non-human tissue culture and then inactivating these by using heat or chemicals. The inactivated pathogens, although weakened, challenge the host's immune system to generate antibodies.

Since the organisms in an inactivated vaccine have been killed, they cannot replicate. Thus, the entire dose of the antigen needed by the body to produce an effective immune response needs to be administered. Inactivated vaccines are easy to produce and are safe. They cannot cause disease, even in persons with compromised immune systems. Moreover, these vaccines are usually heat stable and do not need exact storage temperatures.

However, inactivated vaccines produce a weak immune response. The immunity also diminishes with time. Therefore, this class of vaccines always needs administration of supplemental doses to boost immunity. Manufacturers add adjuvants to the vaccines to boost the immune response. Currently available inactivated vaccines include Salk's polio vaccine, and rabies, cholera, influenza, typhoid fever, plague, whooping cough, hepatitis A and pertussis vaccines.[28]

A class of inactivated vaccines includes toxoid vaccines, which are made by deactivating altered forms of the toxins by chemical or physical methods. Examples of such vaccines include the tetanus toxoid and diphtheria vaccines.

SUBUNIT VACCINES: A PART OF THE PATHOGEN CAN INDUCE IMMUNITY TOO

In the case of subunit vaccines, instead of the entire pathogen, only its antigenic component is administered to trigger a protective immune response. The components used are polysaccharides or proteins.[29]

Subunit vaccines are preferred when an entire inactivated vaccine is too immunogenic for a host and causes adverse reactions. These vaccines are safe even for immuno-compromised persons and can be made at a low cost in large quantities. However, the immune response is weak and requires the addition of adjuvants and repeated immunization. Examples of subunit vaccines include vaccines for pertussis, hepatitis B, shingles and human papillomavirus (HPV).[30]

Polysaccharide-based vaccines are usually composed of pure bacterial cell wall polysaccharide. Such polysaccharide vaccines are available for pneumococcal disease, meningococcal disease and *Salmonella typhi*. In conjugate polysaccharide vaccines, the polysaccharide is chemically linked to a protein, which makes the vaccine potent. Such vaccines include the *Haemophilus influenzae* type B vaccine.

GENE-BASED VACCINES: A NEW ERA IS UNFOLDING

Gene-based vaccines are the new-generation vaccines. Vaccine antigens are produced by using genetic engineering technology. The genomes of the pathogen are comprehensively screened to identify genes that produce the protein antigens. The relevant gene is then inserted in a harmless organism to produce the antigen. Gene-based vaccines include recombinant vaccines and nucleic acid vaccines.

RECOMBINANT PROTEIN VACCINES

Genetic engineering technology is used to induce harmless microbes to produce proteins or subunits of pathogens. For example, the viral gene of hepatitis B and HPV is inserted into the gene of the yeast cell. The yeast cell so modified produces hepatitis B surface antigen or HPV capsid protein, which is harvested and used as a vaccine. Recombinant vaccines are less reactogenic, safe and potent, and can be used to provide protection against multiple strains of the pathogen.

RECOMBINANT VECTOR VACCINES

Bacterial and viral vector vaccines are developed by genetically engineering a bacterium or a virus to express the gene of interest in order to give genetic instructions to the host cells to produce antigens of the target pathogen in the body to trigger an immune response. The bacteria or the virus used in the vaccine is different from the pathogen the vaccine is targeting. The pathogen in the vaccine is thereby weakened and does not cause disease.

A commonly used virus vector is adenovirus, which causes the common cold. The measles virus, alpha viruses, pox viruses and the vesicular stomatitis virus are also used as vectors. Generally, vector vaccines mimic natural infection and induce a strong immune response, except in people who have pre-existing neutralizing antibodies against the vector due to previous exposure to the pathogen.[31,32] Scientists address this problem by using bacterial or virus vectors to which humans are naïve, for instance, chimpanzee adenoviruses. These vaccines are cheaper than other vaccines and have less stringent storage requirements.

NUCLEIC ACID VACCINES

In this category of jabs, the vaccine shuttles a tiny amount of nucleic acid—either deoxyribonucleic acid (DNA) or ribonucleic acid (RNA)—which is coded for a pathogen-specific antigen, into the host's cell. The cells read the instructions contained in the nucleic acid and replicate copies of the viral or bacterial protein (antigen). The antigens so produced are recognized by the immune system, which produces an immune response to prepare the body to fight the real pathogen.[33]

Nucleic acid vaccines are safe, fast, easy to produce and scale up, and non-infectious. Since the antigen is produced inside our own cells and in large quantities, they induce a strong immune response. However, RNA vaccines need to be stored at ultra-cold temperatures at –70 °C or lower, a challenge in low- and middle-income countries (LMICs). Moreover, there is relatively limited data on the safety and efficacy of these vaccines for humans.

Since the only distinction between nucleic acid vaccines for different pathogens is the sequence of the gene inserted, the manufacturing process of such vaccines is generic in nature. Only the code needs to be changed for different pathogens. Such manufacturing processes are very useful in pandemic situations when vaccines need to be designed, developed and disseminated swiftly.

Nucleic acid vaccines are of two types: RNA vaccines, which use an RNA containing vector delivered using lipid nanoparticles, and DNA vaccines, which use a genetically engineered plasmid DNA to deliver the desired genetic sequence to the cells.[34]

DEVELOPING A VACCINE: INVESTMENT OF MANY YEARS AND MILLIONS OF DOLLARS

Development of a vaccine is a difficult, complex, lengthy, expensive and risky process. It involves a linear sequence of steps over many years. End-to-end development of a vaccine may take more than 10 years and cost up to $500 million.[35] Moreover, all vaccine candidates do not convert to licensed vaccines, which makes the development of a vaccine a risky business.[36] There are five stages required to take a vaccine from a laboratory to people.

Stage 1: Discovery Research

Vaccine development begins with the lengthy process of research in a laboratory to identify a viable vaccine candidate. Researchers look for antigens that will trigger an immune response. Antigens include substances that are derived from germs such as viral capsids, virus-like particles and modified bacterial toxins. This phase normally takes between two and five years and may lead to the discovery of a promising vaccine candidate.

Stage 2: Pre-clinical Studies

Promising vaccine candidates are further evaluated for safety and efficacy by testing them on animals. Usually, mice or monkeys are used for this. At this stage, the vaccine is tested for its toxicity and to assess how the body reacts to it. Testing leads to determination of a safe dose of the vaccine for human trials. At this stage, there is an investigation on whether the vaccine candidate produces a strong enough immune response. This stage may take up to two years. Many vaccine candidates are not successful at the start of the preclinical stage, but some cross this hurdle.

Stage 3: Clinical Trials

Vaccine candidates that emerge victorious at Stage 2 move to the clinical stage. Clinical trials are research studies that determine whether a new vaccine is safe and effective in humans and to calibrate the right dosage. Researchers judge the efficacy of the vaccine and look for adverse events or unwanted side effects in people who take it. For this, the vaccine is tested on humans in three phases.[37]

In Phase 1 clinical trials, the vaccine candidate is administered to a small number of healthy people (between 20 and 200). These trials are carried out over a few months to two years and focus on detecting serious side effects. The success of a trial moves the vaccine candidate to Phase 2 clinical trials.

Phase 2 clinical trials further explore the safety of a vaccine candidate and also start exploring its efficacy. At this phase, the vaccine is administered to a few hundred volunteers as well as to people at risk of contracting the disease. Volunteers are often divided randomly into two groups. One group gets the vaccine and the other group, called the placebo or control group, doesn't. The consistency of the immune response and strength of the immune response to the dose decided at Phase 1 are assessed, and the side effects, if any, are noted. The phase takes two to three years. Phase 2 trials determine the best dose for effectiveness and safety and the right number of doses.

Only a few vaccine candidates make it to the Phase 3 clinical trial stage. This phase aims at determining how effective the vaccine is at preventing the disease and the kind of immune reaction it triggers. Adverse events after vaccination and rare side effects that only show up in a large group are also monitored. Thousands of volunteers are needed for this phase of the clinical trial, which takes several years and generates robust data on the efficacy and safety of the vaccination. Volunteers are randomly divided into two groups, one of which gets the vaccine while the other gets a placebo. Vaccines that do well in this phase move to the licensure stage.

Stage 4: Regulatory Approval

After completion of Phase 3 clinical trials, the vaccine developers submit data and information on the efficacy and safety of the vaccine candidate to the regulatory authority of the country. The regulatory authority reviews the data and information submitted and takes a decision regarding grant of license. A vaccine is only licenced after it has met rigorous standards of efficacy and safety, and when its potential benefits in preventing the disease outweigh the associated risks. The process may take one to two years. Once approval is received, the vaccine is ready for marketing for general use.

Stage 5: Post-marketing Surveillance

Even the largest prelicensure trials may be inadequate to assess a vaccine's potential to induce possible rare or long-term side effects. Therefore, even after licensure, it is essential to keep monitoring vaccine-associated adverse events for years. Changes in the vaccine's effectiveness are also monitored.

HERD IMMUNITY: A COLLECTIVE FORCE TO DEFEAT A CONTAGION

An infectious disease cannot be eliminated or effectively controlled till sufficient numbers of people in the community are vaccinated. This process is called achieving 'herd immunity'. Community immunity or herd immunity occurs when a large proportion of the population has developed immunity against a pathogen, making it difficult for the pathogen to spread. This is because when a high percentage of the population becomes immune, the pathogen cannot pass from one person to another. This breaks the chain of infection and effectively stops a disease from circulating.

Community or herd immunity is also important because it protects people, especially those who are not vaccinated due to their vulnerability, for example, immune-compromised people, babies and the elderly. The minimum percentage of people that need to be vaccinated for an infectious disease to reach herd immunity varies. Highly infectious diseases need a larger proportion of immune people to reach herd immunity. For example, in measles, 95 per cent of the population needs to be vaccinated to attain herd immunity.[35]

A SNEAK PEEK AT THE BOOK

This book presents the 225 years' journey of vaccines from the Jennerian era to the COVID-19 pandemic from an Indian perspective. It's a journey that is characterized by victories against several infectious diseases such as smallpox, polio, rabies and measles. The book also aims to satisfy the curiosity about vaccines that has emerged in the backdrop of the ongoing fight against COVID-19 pandemic.

The book is divided into nine chapters, each presenting an important facet of vaccines to the readers. The epilogue, the final piece, delves into lessons learnt so far and the challenges ahead. It also introduces details of new-generation vaccines including therapeutic vaccines. Finally, it talks about new vistas for the growth of the Indian vaccine industry and how it can do better.

Apart from stories of the evolution of vaccines in the first two chapters and their diverse economic and social benefits in Chapter 4, this book presents many new facets of vaccines. Vaccines are being used by countries to increase their soft power, cement and deepen their ties with other countries, get a foothold in new markets, generate international goodwill and raise their global standing. Consequently, vaccine diplomacy has gained currency in recent times. This includes the 'Vaccine Maitri' initiative launched by India, which is discussed in Chapter 8.

In every era, leadership has been the key force behind the success of vaccines and mass immunization campaigns. In Chapter 9, the book elaborates on this aspect, which traditionally plays a major role in determining the success of this public health weapon. The protective shield of vaccines works the best when everyone is vaccinated. Therefore, vaccine equity, both between and within countries, is critical. Vaccine nationalism, vaccine hoarding and vaccine discrimination crack this basic fabric of public health. Vaccine hesitancy, spurred by lack of trust and misinformation or disinformation spread by anti-vax is another formidable challenge about which this book talks in Chapter 7.

The COVID-19 pandemic has witnessed unprecedented international cooperation, scientific innovation, process simplification and financing efforts, leading to the development of a bouquet of vaccines at lightning speed. There is great interest in the healthcare and its allied sectors to know how this was made possible. This book tries to answer the queries in Chapter 5.

The world's story of vaccines is incomplete without India, which has earned the reputation of being a 'vaccine superpower'. Chapter 3 tells the story of India's evolution in the world's vaccine arena. India's cost-effective vaccines are now supplied to almost every country in the world. And India has not only gifted the world three COVID-19 vaccines in record time but has also successfully carried out the world's largest vaccination drive. This has generated tremendous hope and excitement in people. Chapter 6 reveals many interesting facets of the world's largest vaccination drive undertaken by India to fight COVID-19.

This book is a tribute to our dedicated scientists, public health leaders, frontline health workers, entrepreneurs and countless human beings who have devoted their entire lives to discover and sharpen the power of vaccine arsenals. Their untiring efforts and unwavering commitment have provided a reprieve to humanity from innumerable infectious diseases.

REFERENCES

1. Merriam-Webster's Word of the Year 2021 [Internet]. www.merriam-webster.com. 2021 [cited 26 December 2021]. Available from: https://www.merriam-webster.com/words-at-play/word-of-the-year/vaccine
2. Word of the year 2021: Two iterations of 'vaccine', NFT amongst word of the year chosen by top dictionaries [Internet]. www.indiatoday.in. 2021 [cited 26 December 2021]. Available from: https://www.indiatoday.in/

education-today/grammar-vocabulary/story/word-of-the-year-2021-two-iterations-of-vaccine-nft-amongst-word-of-the-year-chosen-by-top-dictionaries-1888889-2021-12-17

3. Tahseen I. 'Vaccine' is 2021 word of the year after 601% rise in searches for it! *Times of India* [Internet]. timesofindia.indiatimes.com. 2021 [cited 26 December 2021]. Available from: https://timesofindia.indiatimes.com/life-style/spotlight/vaccine-is-2021-word-of-the-year-after-601-rise-in-searches-for-it/articleshow/88021767.cms#:~:text=The%20year%20end%20is%20here,shot%20up%20601%25%20over%202020
4. Cucinotta D, Vanelli M. WHO declares COVID-19 a pandemic. *Acta Bio Medica: AteneiParmensis*. 2020; 91(1):157.
5. Naming the coronavirus disease (COVID-19) and the virus that causes it [Internet]. Who.int. 2021 [cited 26 December 2021]. Available from: https://www.who.int/emergencies/diseases/novel-coronavirus-2019/technical-guidance/naming-the-coronavirus-disease-(covid-2019)-and-the-virus-that-causes-it
6. COVID-19 Public Health Emergency of International Concern (PHEIC) Global research and innovation forum [Internet]. Who.int. 2021 [cited 26 December 2021]. Available from: https://www.who.int/publications/m/item/covid-19-public-health-emergency-of-international-concern-(pheic)-global-research-and-innovation-forum
7. UK authorises world's first Covid-19 vaccine, Pfizer/BioNTech's BNT162b2 [Internet]. Pharmaceutical-technology.com. 2021 [cited 26 December 2021]. Available from: https://www.pharmaceutical-technology.com/features/pfizer-covid-19-vaccine-approved-uk/
8. Dobson AP, Carper ER. Infectious diseases and human population history. *Bioscience*. 1996 Feb 1;46(2):115–126.
9. Smallpox [Internet]. Who.int. 2021 [cited 26 December 2021]. Available from: https://www.who.int/health-topics/smallpox#tab=tab_1
10. Spinney L. Smallpox and other viruses plagued humans much earlier than suspected. *Nature*. 2020;584(7819):30–32.
11. Mühlemann B, Jones TC, Damgaard PD, Allentoft ME, Shevnina I, Logvin A, Usmanova E, Panyushkina IP, Boldgiv B, Bazartseren T, Tashbaeva K. Ancient hepatitis B viruses from the Bronze Age to the Medieval period. *Nature*. 2018 May;557(7705):418–423.
12. Rasmussen S, Allentoft ME, Nielsen K, Orlando L, Sikora M, Sjögren KG, Pedersen AG, Schubert M, Van Dam A, Kapel CM, Nielsen HB. Early divergent strains of Yersinia pestis in Eurasia 5,000 years ago. *Cell*. 2015 October; 163(3):571–582.
13. Mehndiratta MM, P Mehndiratta, R Pande. Poliomyelitis: historical facts, epidemiology and current challenges in eradication. *The Neurohospitalist*. 2014 October; 4(4):223–229.
14. World Health Organization. Smallpox—Eradicating an ancient scourge in bugs, drugs and smoke: stories from public health. World Health Organization; 2012.

15. Jordan D. The discovery and reconstruction of the 1918 pandemic virus [Internet]. Centers for Disease Control and Prevention. 2021 [cited 26 December 2021]. Available from: https://www.cdc.gov/flu/pandemic-resources/reconstruction-1918-virus.html
16. Bagcchi S. Surviving polio with disabilities. *The Lancet Infectious Diseases.* 2019 March1;19(3):251.
17. Vaccine: The word's history ain't pretty [Internet]. www.merriam-webster.com. 2021 [cited 26 December 2021]. Available from: https://www.merriam-webster.com/words-at-play/vaccine-the-words-history-aint-pretty
18. Baxby D. Edward Jenner's inquiry after 200 years. *BMJ.* 1999 February 6;318(7180):390.
19. Markel H. Science diction: The origin of the word 'vaccine'. Available from: https://www.sciencefriday.com/articles/the-origin-of-the-word-vaccine/
20. Origin of the term vaccination: History of vaccines [Internet]. History of vaccines.org. 2021 [cited 26 December 2021]. Available from: https://www.historyofvaccines.org/content/origin-term-vaccination
21. Berche P. Louis Pasteur: From crystals of life to vaccination. *Clinical Microbiology and Infection.* 2012 October;18:1–6.
22. Louis Pasteur and the development of the attenuated vaccine [Internet]. www.vbivaccines.com. 2021 [cited 26 December 2021]. Available from: https://www.vbivaccines.com/evlp-platform/louis-pasteur-attenuated-vaccine/
23. Rappuoli R, Mandl CW, Black S, De Gregorio E. Vaccines for the twenty-first century society. *Nature Reviews Immunology.* 2011 December;11(12):865–872.
24. Statement of the Twenty-ninth Polio IHR Emergency Committee [Internet]. Who.int. 2021 (cited 26 December 2021). Available from: https://www.who.int/news/item/20-08-2021-statement-of-the-twenty-ninth-polio-ihr-emergency-committee
25. Bhatia R. The quest continues for the perfect COVID-19 vaccine. *The Indian Journal of Medical Research.* 2021 January;153(1–2):1.
26. FAQ [Internet]. Icmr.org. 2021 [cited 26 December 2021]. Available from: https://vaccine.icmr.org.in/
27. Bhatia R. The quest continues for perfect COVID-19 vaccine. *The Indian Journal of Medical Research.* January 2021.153(1–2):1.
28. Jain S, Venkataraman A, Wechsler ME, Peppas NA. Messenger RNA-based vaccines: Past, present, and future directions in the context of the COVID-19 pandemic. Advanced Drug Delivery Reviews. 1 2021 December;179:114000.
29. Vartak A, Sucheck SJ. Recent advances in subunit vaccine carriers. *Vaccines.* 2016 June;4(2):12.
30. Monslow MA, Elbashir S, Sullivan NL, Thiriot DS, Ahl P, Smith J, Miller E, Cook J, Cosmi S, Thoryk E, Citron M. Immunogenicity generated by mRNA vaccine encoding VZV gE antigen is comparable to adjuvanted subunit vaccine and better than live attenuated vaccine in nonhuman primates. *Vaccine.* 2020 August 10; 38(36):5793–5802.

31. Rajão DS, Pérez DR. Universal vaccines and vaccine platforms to protect against influenza viruses in humans and agriculture. *Frontiers in Microbiology*. 2018 February 6;9:123.
32. Callaway E. The race for coronavirus vaccines: A graphical guide. *Nature*. 2020:576–577.
33. Jeyanathan M, Afkhami S, Smaill F, Miller MS, Lichty BD, Xing Z. Immunological considerations for COVID-19 vaccine strategies. *Nature Reviews Immunology*. 2020 October;20(10):615–632.
34. Buchy P, Buisson Y, Cintra O, Dwyer DE, Nissen M, de Lejarazu RO, Petersen E. COVID-19 pandemic: Lessons learned from more than a century of pandemics and current vaccine development for pandemic control. *International Journal of Infectious Diseases*. 2021 November;112:300–317.
35. Frequently asked questions of health care workers [Internet]. www.mohfw.gov.in. 2021 [cited 26 December 2021]. Available from: https://www.mohfw.gov.in/pdf/FAQsforHCWs&FLWs.pdf
36. Lurie N, Saville M, Hatchett R, Halton J. Developing Covid-19 vaccines at pandemic speed. *New England Journal of Medicine*. 2020 May 21;382(21):1969-73.
37. Vaccine FAQs [Internet]. LSHTM. 2021 [cited 26 December 2021]. Available from: https://www.lshtm.ac.uk/research/centres/vaccine-centre/vaccine-faqs

Acknowledgements

At the outset, I would like to thank my gurus, Professor John Porter and Dr Phil Edwards. As my supervisors for my Doctor of Public Health (DrPH) studies at the London School of Hygiene and Tropical Medicine (LSHTM), with immense patience and perseverance, they equipped me with the required skillsets for research writing and motivated me to write.

I would like to express my deepest gratitude to my mentor, an amazing person and a thorough professional, Dr T. V. Somanathan, Finance Secretary, Government of India, for nurturing, protecting, encouraging and guiding me. I would also like to thank Mr Rajesh Bhushan, Secretary, Health and Family Welfare, Government of India, and Ms S. Aparna, Secretary Pharmaceuticals, Government of India, for providing me guidance and sharing with me immensely valuable input.

I also thank all the officers of the Government of India and various state governments who have provided me diverse and useful insights on India's vaccine growth story. I am indebted to my colleagues in the Department of Expenditure, the Ministry of Finance—Ms Annie George Mathews, Special Secretary, and Mr Sanjay Prasad, Additional Secretary and Ms Debashree Mukherjee, Additional Secretary, the Ministry of Jal Shakti—for providing their solid support in my endeavours.

My heartfelt gratitude to all my dear friends who have been my pillars of strength in the highs and lows I went through while writing this book. Their feedback led to immense improvements.

I am immensely grateful to Ms Namarita Kathait, Associate Commissioning Editor at SAGE, for coming up with the idea of a

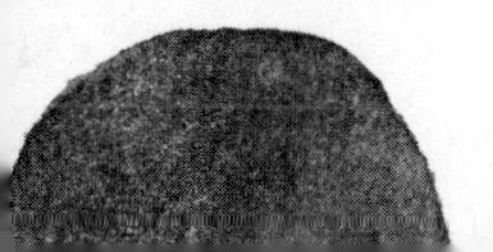

book on this subject and constantly guiding me from inception to completion. Without her, this book would not have seen the light of day. Thank you, Manisha Mathews, Associate Vice President, Commissioning (Books), at SAGE, for taking this book forward to the production stage.

I profoundly thank my wife Sunita, daughter Siya and son Karan, to whom this book is dedicated, for bearing with all the odd hours and efforts that went into this book without complaining. They have been my pillars of strength.

Chapter 1

Cowpox to COVID-19

BIRTH OF FIRST HUMAN VACCINE

It was a pleasant afternoon in June 1765. The market town of Sodbury near Bristol in South Gloucestershire, England, was buzzing with activities. People were busy buying local farm produce and freshly cooked meals. Children were joyfully playing corn hole, quoits, croquet and lawn scrabble.

At the same time, a young girl was visiting Daniel Ludlow, a surgeon and apothecary, with a complaint of fever and rashes on her hands.[1]

While the two were discussing the symptoms of her disease, she told the doctor that she would never have an ugly pockmarked face.

'How?' the doctor asked her with a puzzled look.

'Because I shall never have smallpox,' the girl giggled.

'How on earth do you know that?' the doctor asked, amused.

'Because I have contracted cowpox in the dairy where I work and have blisters on my hands,' the girl said convincingly.

Daniel Ludlow did not understand the connection between cowpox and smallpox. With other patients waiting, he let her go after prescribing medicines.

But this brief conversation caught the mind of Edward Jenner, Ludlow's young apprentice, who was assisting the doctor.

After assisting Ludlow for eight years, Jenner started his own practice in the countryside. He heard the folk stories of people who

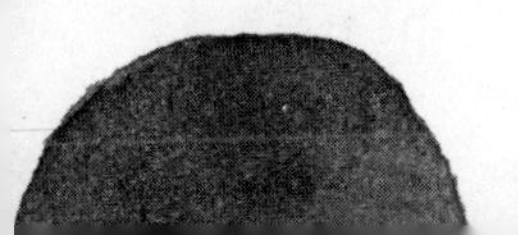

had contracted cowpox getting lifelong protection from smallpox. This was also believed to be the reason for the unblemished complexions of dairymaids.[2]

Cowpox was a mild disease of the cows. It caused a few weeping spots (pox) on their udders. People got infected either from cows or from other people suffering from the disease. Symptoms included mild fever, body ache and a small number of pox, usually on the hands.

The sheer number of stories he heard and the cases he saw prompted Jenner to hypothesize that cowpox protects against smallpox. He postulated that cowpox could be transmitted from one person to another.[3] He decided to test his hypotheses and identified volunteers for his first experiment. They included a dairymaid called Sarah Nelms, who came to him with a cowpox pustule on her hand, and an eight-year-old orphan boy called James Phipps.

Sarah had contracted cowpox from Blossom, a mahogany-brown Gloucester cow. After the success of Jenner's experiment, Blossom became a historical creature. Her portrait was seen in the Jenner Museum in Berkeley at Gloucestershire. After she died, her hide was displayed on the wall of the library of St George's Hospital in London.

On 14 May 1796, Jenner extracted some fluid from a fresh cowpox lesion on Sarah's hand and inoculated it into Phipps's arm. The inoculation was performed by Jenner making two superficial incisions, each about half an inch in length, on Phipps's arm. A couple of days after the inoculation, the boy developed a few pustules and mild fever. He recovered from the illness by the tenth day.

To test his hypothesis, Jenner again inoculated Phipps, but this time with matter from a fresh smallpox lesion, on 1 July 1796. He observed the boy for a few days. To his great relief, Phipps did not develop the disease.[4]

Thus, the world's first vaccine was born. The procedure was called 'vaccination', a term coined by Richard Dunning with Jenner's approval in 1800 (from Latin *vacca,* meaning cow).

A WIFE ENSURES THAT THE WORLD KNOWS HER HUSBAND'S FEAT

A gravestone in a small village called Yetminster in North Dorset, England, reads, 'The first person (known) who introduced the cow-pox inoculation.' However, this is the grave of Benjamin Jesty and not Edward Jenner. Who was Jesty?

Jesty was an enterprising farmer and cattle breeder in Yetminster. In 1774, more than two decades before Jenner's discovery of the vaccine, the demon of smallpox had struck Jesty's village.[2] Jesty was worried about his family but believed that he would be safe, since he had had cowpox a few years ago.

Jesty's two dairymaids, Anne Notley and Mary Reade, had also had cowpox. Since then, they were called on more than one occasion to nurse their relatives who were suffering from smallpox, but did not contract the disease.[5]

Therefore, the enterprising farmer took his wife Elizabeth Notley and two sons Robert, aged 3, and Benjamin, aged 2, to Elford's farm near the hamlet of Chetnole. On reaching there, Jesty wasted no time in identifying a cow in the herd that had cowpox lesions on her udder.

Using a stocking needle, Jesty collected fluid from a lesion and injected it into the skin of his wife's arm, just below the elbow. He repeated the procedure on his sons. The trio suffered from inflammation of their arms and fever for a few days but recovered soon.[2] And they remained unharmed by the smallpox epidemic that ravaged the area. The boys were later injected with smallpox matter from a smallpox pustule by Trowbridge in 1789 but showed no symptoms.[2]

Jesty's paramount interest was in protecting his family. He showed no inclination to publish his results or promote his findings. However, Elizabeth wanted the world to know her husband's contribution.

Hence, she made it a point to engrave his achievements on his tomb.[6]

WORLD BRUSHES ASIDE INDIA'S CLAIM

Did India discover the smallpox vaccine before Edward Jenner?

If we go by what was found by a British officer posted in North India, the answer is 'yes'. In response to an advertisement published in the *Calcutta Gazette* on 7 July 1803 by John Schoolbred, Mr Gillman, a surgeon in the 8th Regiment Native Infantry, had found some pages of a Sanskrit work entitled *Sudhasangraha*. It was composed by a physician called Mahadeva, who had worked under the patronage of Raja Sinha. The text revealed that cowpox vaccine was used to provide protection against *Masurica* (smallpox) and that the practice was in vogue at least a hundred years before Jenner's discovery. The inoculation procedure described in the text had great similarities with Jenner's vaccination process.[7]

However, the veracity of what was claimed in the *Sudhasangraha* was not proved, and the Indian claim has not been taken seriously by the world till today.

THE MOST TERRIBLE OF THE MINISTERS OF DEATH

In ancient times, smallpox was the scourge of humankind. Frequent smallpox epidemics swept across the world, decimating populations. The 'speckled monster' blinded one-third of its survivors and cursed almost all its victims with disfiguring scars.[8] The historian Macaulay has called smallpox 'the most terrible of all the ministers of death'.[9]

The exact origin of smallpox is unknown. The disease is believed to have first appeared in China's agricultural settlements, Indus Valley or Northeast Africa around 3,000 years ago.[9] The earliest evidence of smallpox, like skin lesions, was found on three Egyptian mummies dating 1570 BC to 1085 BC.[8]

Bishop Marius of Avenches used the word 'variola' for the first time to describe the disease (from the Latin word *varius* meaning 'strained', or *varus*, meaning 'mark on the skin') in 570 AD. The term 'small pokes' was first used in England towards the end of the 15th century (from *pocke*, meaning *sac*).[10]

THE INDIAN PLAGUE

Smallpox is believed to have been widely prevalent in India in early times. Some historians and physicians have referred to smallpox as the 'Indian plague'.[11] The disease is also believed to have struck Alexander's army in the Indus Valley in 327 BC.[12]

Other scholars and historians believe that smallpox was introduced in India in the 1st millennium BC by Egyptian traders. However, the earliest recorded epidemic of the disease in India dates back to 1545 AD in Goa. It was most likely introduced by the Portuguese and claimed the lives of 8,000 children.[6,13]

POX ANTIDOTES: SHELTER OF THE DIVINE

Was it only in India that people worshipped the goddess of smallpox, Sheetala?

It was not only in India, but people all over the world also believed that the disease was a punishment from gods and goddesses. Therefore, propitiation of smallpox gods, goddesses and saints was universal.

The Chinese worshipped T'ou-Shen Niang-Niang, the goddess of smallpox. During the middle ages in Europe, St Nzcazse, the

Bishop of Rheims, was revered as the patron saint of smallpox. Tarnetorno received this honour in Japan in the 12th century. Sopona, also called Obafuqe (King of the Earth) or Omofu, was a smallpox deity in Africa.[12]

VARIOLATION: THE ANCIENT WEAPON AGAINST THE SPECKLED MONSTER

Since 430 BC, people have believed that contracting smallpox provided lifelong protection against the disease.[7] This led to the introduction of the practice of variolation (from the Latin word *variola,* meaning smallpox).

In variolation, a tiny amount of material from the pustules of a person infected with smallpox was administered to a healthy individual to prevent a natural infection. It caused mild symptoms of smallpox in the recipient and did not leave scars on the face.[14]

Extensive literature about smallpox has been unable to pinpoint the exact beginning of variolation. However, there is evidence that inoculation against smallpox was practised in India and China around 1000 AD.[15,16]

INDIAN FIGHT AGAINST SMALLPOX WITH *TIKAH*

In one spring in early 18th century a child was crying loudly as his father held him tight. Two cuts had been made on his arm by a middle-aged man popularly called *tikadar* (inoculator). A priest was loudly chanting *mantras* praising the goddess Sheetala, the deity for smallpox.

The *tikadar* opened a bag tied around his waist and rubbed a piece of cotton in a powdery substance in the bag. Then he sprinkled a few drops of *gangajal* (water from the Ganga) on the cotton and divided it into two pieces. The cuts were then covered with the pieces of the cotton.

This was the process of inoculation or *tikah* against smallpox which was prevalent in India a few centuries ago. It is believed that from India, the practice of preventive inoculation spread to China and other countries.[17]

It is believed that the practice of variolation, locally known as *tikah*, was common in India as early as the 16th century. The inoculators were Brahmins. They carried dried pus from previous years' infections and introduced it into the skin of a patient. Groups of tikadars (inoculators) would embark on their journeys every year, during the spring season.

The preferred location for inoculation was the arm, midway between the shoulder and elbow. William Ward, in his book *A View of the History, Literature, and Mythology of the Hindoos,* writes that the parents employed a Brahmin priest to worship Sheetala, the presiding goddess of smallpox, at the time of inoculation, and as the disease progressed.[18]

The British took the practice to South India.[19] In 1787, Surgeon Nicol Mein variolated 20 European troops in Trichinopoly.

INSUFFLATION: THE CHINESE METHOD OF INOCULATION

In 1661, the Emperor of China Fu-lin succumbed to smallpox. Surprisingly, his third son was appointed his successor, ignoring his elder brothers. Why?

This child named K'ang was crowned only because he had survived smallpox and was thus protected for the rest of his life. His elder brothers were yet to face the smallpox demon.

Emperor K'ang became an ardent advocate of smallpox variolation. He got his children and later his troops inoculated. He also wrote a letter to his descendants advocating the virtues of variolation.

It is not known when the practice of variolation commenced in China. However, the book written by Chinese doctor Zhang Lu in 1695 is considered the first available record, which described variolation in China.[20]

According to the vintage Chinese medical text, *The Golden Mirror of Medicine*, written in 1742, four methods of variolation were prevalent in China since 1695—applying smallpox scab powder on cotton wool and inserting it into the nose of a patient, blowing scab powder into the nose, putting on the undergarments of an infected child on a healthy child for several days and stuffing their nose with a piece of cotton smeared with the contents of a vesicle.[21]

Another known method of variolation was making pills of the powder obtained by grinding white cow fleas and administering these orally.[21]

PRESERVING THE BEAUTY QUOTIENT OF IMPERIAL HAREMS

Smallpox inoculation was introduced in Egypt by the Mamelukes in the 13th century. However, it was used largely to preserve the youth of women in the imperial harems, instead of using it on a larger scale to mitigate the severity of smallpox in the community.[12] It made its way to Turkey from Egypt.

According to Dr Emanuel Timoni, innoculation against smallpox was introduced in Constantinople by Circassians, Georgians and other Asiatics.[14] Others posit that the practice was brought to Constantinople via the Sublime Porte to the Ottoman Empire in 1670 by Caucasian women from the Caucasus. These women, who were famous for their legendary beauty, were in great demand in the harems of Turkish sultans. Many of these women were inoculated in those parts of their bodies where their scars would not be seen.[3] The methods of variolation used in India and in the Ottoman Empire were similar, pointing towards their common origin.

According to Cassem Algaida Aga, who was the ambassador to the Court of St James from Tripoli, inoculation was being practised by Arabs in North Africa even before 1700.[22] Aga had been inoculated along with his four brothers and three sisters in his childhood.

Lady Mary Wortley Montague: Ambassador of Variolation from Europe

Lady Mary Wortley Montague was the wife of Sir Edward Wortley Montague, the ambassador of the United Kingdom to the Sublime Porte. She had contracted smallpox in 1715. This had disfigured her beautiful face.

When she arrived in the Ottoman Empire two years later, she was happy to learn about the practice of variolation. She was very eager to protect her children from the curse.

Lady Montague asked Dr Charles Maitland, the embassy surgeon, to inoculate her five-year-old son, Edward. Maitland arranged for the procedure, which was performed on 18 March 1778 at Pera near Constantinople.

After the return of the Montague family to the United Kingdom, at Lady Montague's request, Maitland inoculated her four-year-old daughter in April 1721. This was the first professional variolation procedure and was also the first procedure to be performed in England. The process was carried out in the presence of the physicians of the royal court.[3] To promote variolation, Mary later took her daughter to the homes of smallpox patients to demonstrate her immunity. Although this aroused interest in inoculation, there was still hesitance. People were waiting for some more experiments.

Royal clinical trials

Do you know that the first human trial of variolation in Europe were conducted on prisoners and orphans?

It was organized at the behest of Caroline, the Princess of Wales. The venue of the first one was Newgate prison, which is located at the corner of Newgate Street and Old Bailey Street in London.

The 'Newgate Guinea Pigs' were six condemned criminals who were assured of the royal pardon if they submitted to the experiment. These criminals included three women, Mary North, Ann Tompion and Elizabeth Harrison, aged 19–36 years, and three men, John Cauthrey, John Allcock and Richard Evans, aged 19–25 years.[20] They were granted conditional pardons on 4 July 1721 and were reprieved on 21 July 1721.

The prisoners were inoculated by Charles Maitland on 9 August 1721. A distinguished crowd of court physicians, members of the Royal Society and of the College of Physicians were in attendance. The prisoners survived the procedure and were later found to be immune to smallpox.[23]

The next experiment was conducted on five orphans from St James' Parish in Westminster in March 1722.[24] It proved that variolation was safe and resulted in a mild case of smallpox and immunity to it in the future.[20]

Royalty were convinced to take the inoculations. In April 1722, Maitland inoculated Amelia and Caroline, the granddaughters of the King and daughters of the Princess of Wales.[25]

The College of Physicians declared its unqualified support of variolation in 1755.The procedure soon gained popularity in England and also spread to other countries in Europe.[26]

A SLAVE TEACHES INOCULATION TO AMERICA

It was a sunny noon on a day in March 1714. Mercury had started rising in Boston. Rev Cotton Mather, a congregational minister in Boston, was looking at his slave Onesimus in disbelief. The slave, who was from Garamantee, had just told him that he was fully protected against smallpox. On further enquiry, he told

Mather about the practice of variolation prevalent in his native land for protection against smallpox. But Mather refused to believe him.

A few months later, Mather read Dr Emanuel Timoni's account of variolation in Constantinople, which was published by the Royal Society in its *Philosophical Transactions* in the April–June 1714. Mather decided to confirm the variolation story he heard from Onesimus. He was told that the slaves immune from smallpox could attend smallpox patients.[27]

The arrival of a ship carrying persons infected with smallpox led to an outbreak of smallpox in Boston and other parts of Massachusetts in 1721. Mather decided to try variolation to save the people. He convinced Dr Zabdiel Boylston to inoculate Bostonians.

The drive started on 26 June 1721, with the inoculation of Boylston's six-year-old son and two of his slaves. The first variolation programme in the Americas had begun. Mather and Boylston went on to inoculate 244 people.[28]

Perhaps for the first time, the duo used a comparative analysis method to evaluate their procedure. They compared the mortality rate of people infected by smallpox with those whose illness had been contracted from variolation. They found that only 2 per cent of the variolated persons died, compared to 14 per cent of those who had contracted the disease naturally.[29] The popularity of variolation therefore grew in New England's colonies.

The practice of variolation to protect against smallpox became increasingly popular and continued across the world till Edward Jenner discovered vaccination. This was the beginning of a new world.

VACCINE CLERK TO THE WORLD

After discovering the first vaccine, Jenner spent the rest of his life popularizing his discovery and supplying cowpox material across the world. He was of the view that his discovery was for the global good. He was supported by some other surgeons of his time, such as Henry Cline, Dr William Woodville and Dr George Pearson.

The vaccination process spread with remarkable speed and reached almost all the European countries.[4] It is estimated that by 1801, the number of persons vaccinated in England rose to 100,000.

Despite supply-related constraints, Jenner sent the vaccine to anyone who requested it. Since he was so involved in corresponding about the vaccine, he used to call himself the 'Vaccine Clerk to the World'.[30]

SPREAD OF JENNER'S VACCINE ACROSS THE WORLD

In 1803, King Charles IV of Spain asked the royal physician Francisco Xavier de Balmis to introduce smallpox vaccination in the Spanish colonies in the New World. Dr Balmis started his expedition on a ship with 22 abandoned children and many assistants. During the journey, he vaccinated the boys in sets of two. This was done to ensure the availability of fresh pustules at any given time. When he reached Caracas, only one of the children had a visible cowpox pustule. However, that was sufficient to initiate vaccination in South America.[6]

Jenner's vaccine travelled across the world through vaccination of children. He had supplied vaccines to Dr John Haygarth who in turn shared some of the material with Professor Benjamin Waterhouse. Waterhouse introduced vaccination in New England. He could convince the city's Board of Health to sponsor a public test of vaccination in 1802 in which 19 volunteers were vaccinated.[31]

In Russia, Empress Dowager became a strong advocate of vaccination. A young orphan was administered the first smallpox vaccine and she named her 'Vaccinoff'. She also provided the girl a pension for life.[6]

SMALLPOX VACCINE ARRIVED IN INDIA

Several attempts were made by Jenner and others to send cowpox vaccine material to India by sea. However, owing to its short shelf life, particularly in hot and humid climates, these attempts were unsuccessful. Jenner also sent some vaccine material to Swiss physician Jean de Carro who sent part of it to Baghdad via Vienna and Constantinople.

In Baghdad, a British surgeon propagated a fresh vaccine for local children, which was carried to India by successive person-to-person inoculations on a ship enroute to Bombay (now Mumbai).[7,32]

On 14 June 1802, the first vaccination of 20 children was carried out in Bombay by Dr Hllenus Scott. However, the pustules developed only in Anna Dusthall, the three-year-old daughter of the female help of a British officer.[33] From the fluid of her pustule, five children were vaccinated. More material was collected and sent to different places, including Poona, Surat, Hyderabad, Ceylon, Madras and places along the coast and the Deccan.

After that, the vaccine was sent to major locations of in British India. A regular official vaccination establishment was created in India in May 1803.[32] Vaccination was soon administered all across British India where European children were inoculated.

Initially, the lymph required for vaccination came from England. It was kept alive through a chain of volunteers. Later, cow farms were established in each Indian state for production of vaccine lymph.

MEETING THE PRODUCTION AND PRESERVATION CHALLENGE

For how long could the arm-to-arm propagation of vaccines be sustained? Was it sufficient to defeat the speckled monster? No, the world needed a larger supply of vaccines and new methods to transport them.

In 1810, Gennaro Galbiati, director of the vaccine service in Naples in Italy, retro vaccinated cows with human vaccine lymph. From the resulting animal lymph, he vaccinated people. Galbiati found that such vaccines manifested their results more quickly, but without being more dangerous or compromising protection compared to humanized viruses. Moreover, vaccines of cow lymph posed no danger of transmitting other human diseases from the donor to the recipient.[6]

Later in 1836, Edward Ballard, an English physician, reached the conclusion that there was a decline in the potency of cowpox virus, which was transmitted from humans to humans. He made two suggestions to overcome this problem. The first was to select new strains of cowpox. In the second method, he suggested boosting the potency to reintroduce the pustule matter (lymph) back into cows. These methods greatly helped in producing sufficient vaccine material.[6]

Cheyne's discovery in the 1850s further strengthened the vaccine supply chain. He found that mixing vaccine lymph with glycerol prevented its decomposition and facilitated prolonged storage of the vaccine. By the end of the 19th century, glycerinated calves' lymph became the standard procedure and arm-to arm-vaccination was stopped. Another milestone in improving the stability of vaccines, especially in tropical areas, was the development of dried vaccine preparations in Germany and France.[9]

CULTIVATING VACCINES IN LABS

Jenner's path-breaking discovery had many limitations. Not many human diseases had a suitable animal analogue capable of conferring immunity without causing the disease. The problem was aggravated by the subsequent realization that a single dose of cowpox matter was not enough to provide lifelong protection.

Therefore, the scientists started working on ways to grow pathogens in labs and managed to strip them of their power to make the recipients sick. However, the capability of stimulating the immune system to recognize a virus in the event of an actual infection and neutralize it was not compromised. In the next chapter, we will know more about the new era of vaccinology—the era of lab-grown vaccines.

REFERENCES

1. Parish HJ. *Victory with vaccines: The story of immunization*. Edinburgh: E&S Livingstone; 1968.
2. Pead PJ. Benjamin Jesty: New light in the dawn of vaccination. *The Lancet*. 2003 December;362(9401):2104–2109.
3. Riedel S. Edward Jenner and the history of smallpox and vaccination. *Baylor University Medical Center Proceedings*. 2005 January 21;18(1):21–25.
4. Willis NJ. Edward Jenner and the eradication of smallpox. *Scottish Medical Journal*. 1997;42:118–121.
5. Brimnes N. Variolation, vaccination and popular resistance in early colonial south India. *Medical History*. 2004 April;48:199–228.
6. The history of vaccines [Internet]. History of vaccines.org. 2021 [cited 17 May 2021]. Available from: https://www.historyofvaccines.org/timeline#EVT_30
7. Wujastyk D. A pious fraud: Indian claims for pre-Jennerian smallpox vaccination. In: Meulenbeld GJ, Wujastyk D, editors. *Studies on Indian medical history*. Delhi: Motilal Banarsidass Publishers; 2001. 121–154.
8. Barquet N, Domingo P. Smallpox: The triumph over the most terrible of the ministers of death. *Ann Intern Med*. 1997;127(8 Pt 1):635–642.
9. World Health Organization. The global eradication of smallpox: Final report of the Global Commission for the Certification of Smallpox Eradication, Geneva, December 1979. World Health Organization. 1980.
10. Moore JC. *The history of smallpox*. London: Longman; 1815.
11. Lahariya C. A brief history of vaccines and vaccination in India. *The Indian Journal of Medical Research*. 2014 April;139(4):491.
12. Fenner F, Henderson DA, Arita I, Jezek Z, Ladnyi ID. The history of smallpox and its spread around the world. *Smallpox and Its Eradication*. 1988. 209–244.
13. Banthia J, Dyson T. Smallpox in nineteenth-century India. *Population and Development Review*. 1999 December;25(4):649–680.
14. Timonius E. An account of the history of procuring the small pox by incision or inoculation: as it has for some time been practised at Constantinople. Being the extract of a letter from Emanuel Timonius, Oxon and Patav. M.D. F.R.S. December 1713. Constantinople. Phil Trans 1714;29:72–82.
15. Fitchett JR, Heymann DL. Smallpox vaccination and opposition by anti-vaccination societies in 19th century Britain. *Hist Med*. 1995;2:E17.

16. Needham J, Lu GD. *Science and civilisation in China, Volume 6, biology and biological technology, Part VI, medicine.* Cambridge: Cambridge University Press; 2000.
17. Dharampal S (editor). *Indian science and technology in the eighteenth century: Some contemporary accounts.* Hyderabad: Academy of Gandhian Studies; 1971.
18. Ward WA. *View of the history, literature, and mythology of the Hindoos: Including a minute description of their manners and customs, and translations from their principal works.* Serampore: Printed at the Mission Press; 1818.
19. Bhattacharya S, Harrison M, Worboys M. *Fractured states: Smallpox, public health and vaccination policy in British India*, 1800–1947. Hyderabad: Orient Longman; 2006.
20. Boylston A. The origins of inoculation. *Journal of the Royal Society of Medicine.* 2012 July;105(7):309–313.
21. Plotkin SA Plotkin SA, Orenstein W, Offit PA. *Vaccines.* Amsterdam: Elsevier Health Sciences; 2008.
22. Cassem Algaida Aga Paper relating to the inoculation of smallpox, as it is practised in the Kingdoms of Tripoli, Tunis and Algier. In: Scheuchzer JG, editor. *An account of the success of inoculating the smallpox in Great Britain, for the Years 1727 and 1728.* London: J. Peele; 1729. 61–63.
23. Stearns RP. Remarks upon the introduction of inoculation for smallpox in England. *Bull Hist Med.* 1950;24:103–122.
24. Miller G. Smallpox inoculation in England and America: A reappraisal. *The William and Mary Quarterly.* 1956;13:476–492.
25. Woodville W. *The history of inoculation of the smallpox, in Great Britain.* Vol. 1. London: James Philips; 1796.
26. Kochhar R. Smallpox in the modern scientific and colonial contexts 1721–1840. *Journal of biosciences.* 2011 December 1;36(5):761–768.
27. Mather C. *An account of the method and success of inoculating the small-pox in Boston in New England.* London: J. Peels; 1722.
28. Gross CP, Sepkowitz KA. The myth of the medical breakthrough: smallpox, vaccination and Jenner reconsidered. *Int J Infect Dis.* 1998;3:54–60.
29. Beall OT, Shryock RH. *Cotton Mather: First significant figure in American medicine.* Baltimore: Johns Hopkins University Press; 1954.
30. Zakir F, Islam F, Jabeen A, Moni SS. Vaccine development: A historical perspective. *Biomedical Research.* 2019;30:452–455.
31. Underwood EA. Edward Jenner, Benjamin Waterhouse and the introduction of vaccination in the United States. *Nature.* 1949;163:823–828.
32. Shoolbred J. *Report on the progress of vaccine inoculation in Bengal.* London: Blacks and Perry; 1805.
33. Behbehani AM. The smallpox story: Life and death of an old disease. *Microbiol. Rev.* 1983;47:455–509.

Chapter 2

Evolution of Vaccines

A MISTAKE LEADING TO A PHENOMENAL DISCOVERY

The French chemist and microbiologist, Louis Pasteur, was seething with anger. He was just back from his summer vacation in 1879. His assistant, Charles Chamberland, had ignored his instructions and had not inoculated the chicken with the cholera bacilli as he had been directed.

Pasteur was studying the progression of fowl cholera by injecting a chicken with the live bacteria, *Pasteurella multocida*. To cool down his boss's temper, Chamberland immediately inoculated the chicken. Both he and Pasteur expected that the chicken would die in a few days, as usual. However, to his and Pasteur's surprise, the chicken showed only mild symptoms of the disease and recovered. They thought that the culture had gone bad and injected the recovered chicken with a fresh culture of bacteria, but to their astonishment, the chicken showed no signs of the disease.[1]

Pasture hypothesized that exposure to oxygen for a prolonged period had weakened the bacteria without affecting their ability to induce immunity.

There was this striking similarity to the weakened smallpox virus in the old pus used by Indian *teekadars* for protection against smallpox, but by then the world had moved close to the production of vaccines in laboratories.

FIRST PUBLIC DEMONSTRATION OF ATTENUATED VACCINE

5 May 1881: A Momentous Day

In a small French village called Pouilly-le-Fort, a huge crowd had gathered at the farm of Monsieur Rossignol—government officials, farmers, journalists, local leaders and scientists. Everyone was vying to get a fuller view of the first ever demonstration of a lab-grown vaccine.[2]

Monsieur De la Rochette, president of the Agriculture Society of Melun, had arranged more than 60 animals for the experiment. Louis Pasteur arrived with his attenuated anthrax vaccine. Caused by *bacillus anthracis,* anthrax can affect both humans and animals. However, the disease was more common among livestock and caused huge economic losses on account of death and loss of productivity.[3]

Pasteur divided the animals into two groups—the 'experiment group' and the 'control group', with each group having 24 sheep, 6 cows and 1 goat. The experiment group was inoculated with attenuated anthrax bacilli, while 'control group' was not inoculated.[2]

The experiment group was re-inoculated on 17 May 1881 with a more virulent but still attenuated bacillus. The crowd assembled again on 31 May 1881. This time, both the experiment group and the control group were challenged with a virulent anthrax bacillus. The spectators were asked to come back after 48 hours to see the results.[2]

The spectators were astonished when they arrived at the farm on 2 June 1881—21 sheep and the goat in the control group' were dead. All the animals in the experiment group were healthy.[2]

Two more sheep in the control group died soon in front of the crowd. The last sheep in this group was also dead at the end of the day, and although the cows in the control group did not die, they showed clear symptoms of the disease.[2]

The world was then convinced of the potency of cultivated vaccines.

SNATCHED FROM THE JAWS OF DEATH

A desperate mother from Alsace in France was looking for Louis Pasteur. She had heard rumours that he was working on a cure for the deadly disease, rabies. On 4 July 1885, her nine-year-old son, Joseph Meister, was bitten 14 times by a rabid dog. There was hardly any hope of his survival.

Fortunately, she found a doctor, Dr Joseph Grancher, who knew Pasteur. At her repeated requests, the doctor accompanied the lady to Pasteur's laboratory. Pasteur was convinced by Dr Grancher that Meister's death was imminent and that trying a rabies vaccine, which Pasteur was developing, on him was justified to save his life.[4]

Reluctantly, at 8 PM on 6 July, 1885 Pasteur administered the first rabies vaccine to Meister. It was made from the spinal cord of a rabbit who had died of rabies, air dried for 15 days. Meister was administered the vaccine every day for the next 13 days, but it was made of progressively fresher and thus more virulent spinal cords.[5] This brought back Meister from the clutches of death.

A couple of months later, another boy, Jean Baptiste Jupille, received the same course of treatment and survived the deadly pathogen. The weapon to neutralize another killer pathogen was then on the block.[5]

Pasteur proposed that, in honour of Edward Jenner, the protective procedure should be generally referred to as vaccination.[6]

Later, in 1946, Hilary Koprowsky grew a rabies strain in chicken embryos instead of in nervous system tissues and attenuated it by passing it 180 times through chicken embryos. He called it the high-egg passage (HEP). This virus strain would have fewer side effects and vaccine failures.[7]

A SCIENTIST AND A GUINEA PIG

There was a spectacular scene in the Kattal Bagan *bustee* (slum) on the outskirts of Calcutta in March 1894.

In the midst of small mud houses clustered around a pond, poor people were waiting to get a miraculous injection. They believed this would save them from the deadly disease of cholera.[8]

A young white man sitting by an oil lamp, had been busy vaccinating people since early morning. Several Indian doctors were also in attendance. The white man was John Haffkine.[8]

John Haffkine had developed the cholera vaccine while working at the famous Pasteur Institute in Paris. Although he was employed as a librarian there, he experimented in the bacteriology lab when he was free. He produced a strengthened or 'exalted' culture of cholera bacilli by passing them 39 times through the peritoneal cavity of pigs. Then he attenuated a part of the culture by using heat. His vaccine was administered in two doses. The first one, the attenuated bacteria, was followed by the exalted culture, a few days later.[9]

On 18 July 1892, Haffkine's discovery created a stir in the newspapers and in academic circles. To prove that his preparation was safe, he performed the first human test of the vaccine on himself. Later, he vaccinated six of his colleagues. All of them recovered after a brief bout of fever and local swelling.[10]

After these initial tests, Haffkine needed a place that was rife with cholera to conduct large-scale human trials. In 1893, Lord Frederick Dufferin, a former Viceroy of India who was the British ambassador in Paris, suggested that he go to Bengal in India.

An outbreak of cholera in Kattal Bagan *bustee* provided Haffkine with an ideal proving ground for his nascent vaccine. Over a few days, he inoculated 116 people. In the next couple of months, his team observed 10 cases of cholera in the bustee of which seven were fatal. To Haffkine's satisfaction, all the fatalities were reported from the un-inoculated group. Thus, the Haffkine vaccine was the first effective prophylactic vaccine for a bacterial disease in human beings.[8]

History was made with the first-ever successful clinical trials of a vaccine on Indian soil.

INDIA DEVELOPS ITS FIRST VACCINE

In September 1896, plague was raging in Bombay's tightly packed slums. It had travelled from British Hong Kong on a merchant ship. When the situation became alarming, the governor turned to Haffkine for help and tasked him with developing the world's first plague vaccine.

Haffkine promptly travelled to Bombay and worked tirelessly in a one-room laboratory with the bare minimum staff. He was ready with the vaccine in a record time of three months. On 10 January 1897, in his signature style, he demonstrated the efficacy of the vaccine on himself. Despite his administering 10cc by an injection (against the proposed dose of 3cc), Haffkine recovered after suffering from a severe fever for a few days. He was then ready for human trials.[11]

In the last week of January 1897, a trial was conducted on the inmates of the Byculla House of Correction: 147 inmates were inoculated, and 172 were left untreated. Subsequently, 12 cases of plague and six deaths were recorded in the jail, all among the un-inoculated group.[8]

The success of the trials created a huge demand for the vaccine. Within a year, hundreds of thousands of people were inoculated, saving an innumerable number of human lives.

RISE AND FALL FROM GRACE

Do you know why the Nobel laureate Ronald Ross accused the British of 'disregard for science' and being guilty of 'gross ingratitude to one of its greatest benefactors'? The reason was the injustice meted out to Haffkine.[12]

Initially, the success of Haffkine's vaccine brought him huge honour. He was knighted by the Queen. In December 1901, he was made director-in-chief of the Plague Research Laboratory in Parel, Bombay. But his fall from grace was on the cards.

In March 1902, 10 people died from Tetanus in Mulkowal village in Punjab after being inoculated with Haffkine's plague vaccine. The cause was identified as contamination of a vial of vaccine prepared at Haffkine's Parel Lab.

An inquiry commission pointed its finger at Haffkine, attributing the incident to a change in the procedure of sterilizing the plague vaccine. The commission concluded that the vial must have gotten contaminated in Haffkine's laboratory. He was dismissed from his position as the director of the Plague lab and asked to proceed on leave.[13]

The findings of the inquiry commission were made public in 1906. Haffkine got support from W. J. Simpson, a professor at King's College, London after it became public. Simpson strongly argued, with evidence, that the bottle had been contaminated at the incident site in Punjab and not in Haffkine's laboratory. Other prominent scientists, including the Nobel laureate Ronald Ross, also took up Haffkine's cause. They accused the British government of miscarriage of justice.[13]

Finally, Haffkine was exonerated in November 1907 and joined as director-in-chief of the Calcutta Biological Laboratory, but he was barred from carrying out trials. In 1914, Haffkine retired from service at the relatively young age of 55 and left India as a dejected man.

The people of India paid a heavy price for disgracing 'the saviour of mankind'. The plague peaked in India in 1904, killing 1,143,993 people. Many of them could have been saved by Haffkine's vaccine. In 1925, the Indian government named the Parel Laboratory the Haffkine Institute.

VACCINES FROM VENOM

Indian stories dating back to the 7th century talk about a sect of people drinking a small quantity of snake venom to become immune to its effects. This was toxin immunity, which the Western world discovered many centuries later.

In 1890, Emil von Behring and Kitasato reported the presence of antitoxins in the serum of animals who were given low doses of tetanus and diphtheria toxins. When administered the pathogens of these diseases, the animals showed no symptoms of having contracted them. The finding was so spectacular that commercial production of the diphtheria antitoxin began within a year after that.[14]

Since Von Behring had referred to the rabbit serum containing an antitoxin as an 'immune serum', the term 'immunization' was coined for serum containing antitoxins.[15]

Later, in 1907, chemical inactivation of toxins led to the development of toxoids, which were demonstrated to generate long-lasting immunity without side effects.

In 1923, Alexander Glenny and Barbara Hopkins demonstrated that the diphtheria toxin could be transformed into a toxoid by the addition of formalin, which on inoculation produces immunity. Ramon and Christian Zoeller developed a tetanus toxoid in a similar manner and used it in the first human vaccine against tetanus in 1926.[16]

ONE MORE VACCINE TRIAL IN INDIA

In war, microbes kill more than bullets. This was the landmark statement made by Sir William Osler, the Regius Professor of Medicine at Oxford University. These lines were a part of his letter written to the *Times* in August 1914.[17]

Osler advocated compulsory typhoid vaccination for war-bound British troops. His statement was supported by data. At the beginning of the Spanish-American War in 1898, typhoid fever claimed the lives of 1,590 soldiers at five training camps, compared to only 280 deaths on the battlefield during the entire war. Osler also underscored the fact that in the Boer War, more men died of dysentery and typhoid than in action.[18]

The typhoid vaccine was developed by the British pathologist Almroth Wright in 1896. Simultaneously, the German duo of Richard Pfeiffer and Wilhelm Kolle also demonstrated human immunity against typhoid fever after inoculation with killed typhoid bacteria in the same year. Later, in 1909, Frederick F. Russell developed the first US typhoid fever vaccine.[19]

Almroth Wright made untiring efforts to vaccinate the British troops before the Boer War. However, his endeavours were met with tough resistance and he could inoculate only 14,000 volunteers. The results were catastrophic. During the war, the British army reported more than 58,000 cases of typhoid and 9,000 deaths.[20]

There was a dire need for more trials of the typhoid vaccine before its extensive use in the military. India was once again found to be the favourite destination for trials.

Extensive trials were conducted by the Anti-typhoid Committee of the British Army Medical Department between 1904 and 1908, with 24 units of the British Army going to India and Egypt to be inoculated. When compared later, the attack rate of typhoid among the vaccinated was found to be six-fold lower than the attack rate among the non-vaccinated troops, and despite inviting criticism for the method not being scientific, the trial results influenced a positive decision on typhoid vaccination.[21] Thereafter, typhoid vaccination became an important part of military life.

COWS GIFT ANOTHER VACCINE TO MANKIND

Do you have a small, round bubble or scar on the upper side of your arm? This is caused by your reaction to the tuberculosis (Bacillus Calmette-Guérin [BCG]) vaccine, but not all vaccine recipients have this reaction.

In the 1800s, tuberculosis, caused by *mycobacterium tuberculae*, was a widespread and deadly disease. It was responsible for every third death in middle-age groups and every seventh among all ages.

As in smallpox, the pathogen that caused the disease in cows, *mycobacterium bovis,* was considered a potential vaccine candidate for human tuberculosis. In 1904, French researcher Albert Calmette (1863–1933) obtained a strain of this bacteria, isolated from the milk of an infected cow. He and veterinarian Jean-Marie Camille Guérin started attenuating the bacteria at the Pasteur Institute of Lille, France, in 1908.[22] It took them 13 years to produce a strain of *mycobacterium bovis* that would safely confer immunity to an uninfected human being. This was achieved after cultivating 230 generations of the bacillus in beef bile, potatoes and glycerol. Albert Calmette and Jean Marie Camille Guérin selected weaker and weaker versions with each passage.[23]

The final attenuated strain was named BCG. Ultimately, human trials began on 17 July 1921. The vaccine became available for human use six years later. However, they had to wait for two more decades before experts started recognizing BCG as a safe vaccine.[24,25]

TAMING THE CRIPPLER

Poliomyelitis was a dreaded disease that was rampant in the 20th century. It has crippled millions of people across the globe. In the 1930s, several attempts to develop a poliovirus vaccine proved futile. Many of the test subjects died or were left paralysed.[28]

This included Maurice Brodie's poliovirus vaccine, which was developed at New York University, and the live attenuated poliovirus vaccine developed by John Kolmer at Temple University in Philadelphia. Researchers were under attack from the citizens, media and health administration.[29]

However, in 1949, the scientific community was re-energized by the news that John Enders, Thomas Weller and Frederick Robbins of the Harvard Medical School in the USA had successfully developed the Lansing Strain of poliovirus in human embryonic tissues taken from stillborn foetuses. Cultivation of the virus in human embryonic skin and muscle tissue provided scientists with a simple, relatively inexpensive method of producing large quantities of vaccines and dispensed with the requirement of large animal houses for research on polio. It gave the much-needed push for the development of polio vaccines.[30]

Soon, scientists tasted success. In 1950, Koprowski tested a live attenuated strain of poliovirus on humans at the Wistar Institute in Philadelphia. Like John Haffkine, he tested the vaccine on himself.[31]

However, it was Jonas Salk who earned the distinction of being granted the first license for a trivalent formalin-inactivated polio vaccine on 12 April 1955. Before that, he had tested the vaccine on himself, his wife and their three children on 16 May 1953. This was followed by his conducting a trial on 1.3 million children, beginning 25 April 1954.[32]

Jonas Salk's vaccine was a trivalent inactivated polio vaccine (IPV). It was named the Salk vaccine or the IPV. In Salk's memory, the world observes polio day on 24 October every year.

However, despite the successes, the quest for more and easy-to-administer poliovirus vaccines continued. Albert Sabin conducted trials of his live attenuated oral polio vaccine (OPV) on 10 million Soviet children in 1959. The vaccine was licensed on 24 August 1960. Due to its manifold advantages, OPV gradually ousted its rival IPV from immunization programmes.[33]

DO BOOND ZINDAGI KI

Do boond zindagi ki (two drops of life)! It's not very long ago that we heard these golden words from Amitabh Bachchan, India's biggest superstar. They resonated in all Indian parents' heads, driving them to visit the nearest polio vaccination camp with their children in tow.

India's long and aggressive battle against the crippling disease ultimately led to the realization of the dream of a polio-free India. Delhi conducted the first state-wide polio vaccination campaign on 2 October 1994. This was followed by another round in December 1994. The man who led the campaign as Health Minister of Delhi, Dr Harshvardhan, later became the Health Minister of India. *Polio Ravivar* (Polio Sunday) thereafter became a regular feature throughout the country to mobilize people to vaccination camps.[26]

These concerted efforts paid off, and the number of cases started declining rapidly. The last reported case of polio in India was on 13 January 2011. When no case was reported for three consecutive years, the World Health Organization certified India as being polio-free on 27 March 2014, along with other South-East Asian countries.[27]

Now, all but Pakistan and Afghanistan are polio-free, and the dreaded disease is on the verge of eradication. The 'end game' strategies, now under implementation, will soon make poliomyelitis the second disease to be eradicated from the globe after smallpox.

FAILED ATTEMPTS TO FIGHT THE DEADLIEST INFLUENZA WITH A VACCINE

The COVID-19 pandemic has reminded people of the deadliest flu of the 20th century. Also referred to as the 'Spanish flu', it had infected one-third of the world's population in 1918–1919 and killed an estimated 50 million people. This influenza pandemic was caused by the H1N1 virus.

Many scientists unsuccessfully attempted to develop a vaccine to deal with the pandemic. They tried several killed whole-cell bacterial vaccines. These included *haemophilus influenzae, streptococcus, staphylococcus, pneumococcus, and moraxella catarrhalis.* However, they had failed to correctly identify the causative pathogen. The pandemic was caused by a new strain of the Influenza-A virus and not by any bacteria. In the 1930s, it could only be isolated.[34]

Jonas Salk and Thomas Francis led the development of the first influenza vaccine, which was approved in the USA for military use in 1945.[35]

THE GOLDEN AGE OF VACCINOLOGY

In the 20th century, also called the 'golden age of vaccinology', vaccines for a number of diseases emerged in succession. These included Max Theiler's live attenuated yellow fever vaccine in 1936; Pearl Kendrick and Grace Eldering's pertussis (whooping cough) vaccine in 1939; the vaccine developed by Maurice Hilleman for Japanese encephalitis in 1944; Maurice Hilleman's vaccine for adenovirus in the 1960s; John Ender's vaccine for measles in 1963; Maurice Hilleman's vaccine for Mumps in 1967; Maurice Hilleman's vaccine for rubella in 1969; Michiaki Takahashi's vaccine for varicella in the 1970s; Hilleman's vaccine for chickenpox in 1995; Herald Cow's vaccine for typhus in 1993, and the Cincinnati Group's rotavirus vaccine in 1999, followed by its pentavalent oral version in 2006.

The era of multivalent or combined vaccines was ushered in in 1948 with the diphtheria, tetanus and pertussis (DPT) vaccine. The next to follow was the trivalent measles, mumps and rubella (MMR) vaccine in 1971.

The 1970s brought in the era of polysaccharide vaccines. This new approach in vaccine science uses the polysaccharide outer coating of bacteria instead of live or attenuated pathogens. The first one off the block was the meningococcal polysaccharide vaccine, which was licensed on 2 April 1974. The next to be granted a licence was the vaccine against the *haemophilus influenzae* type b (Hib) disease in 1985.[36]

Next came the subunit viral vaccines with the licensing of Hilleman's human-blood-derived hepatitis B vaccine in 1981. Here, instead of a whole virus, a surface protein of the virus was transformed into an effective vaccine. However, there were concerns about HIV infection due to the use of human serum.

This problem was solved by the advent of genetic engineering in vaccine production, which was pioneered by Stanley Cohen and Herbert Boyer. Also referred to as a recombinant technology, it enabled the use of yeast, bacteria, animal cells and insect cells as substrates for the production of immunogenic proteins in 1986. For example, yeast cells were changed so that they produced the protein that was the active ingredient of the hepatitis B vaccine. Later, Hilleman developed the hepatitis A vaccine in a similar manner in 1995. Another subunit vaccine that was licensed in 2006 was the HPV vaccine.

Robbins and Rachel Schneerson ushered in the epoch of conjugate vaccines. They coupled the diphtheria toxoid with the Hib type B capsule. The first in this category was the pneumococcal conjugate vaccine (PCV7) for pneumococcal disease in 2000. Another conjugate vaccine was licensed for meningococcal group A in 2010.

According to the WHO, vaccines are now available for 25 diseases, and vaccines against 15 more pathogens are in the pipeline.[38] However, new pathogens keep emerging to challenge mankind. Vaccinology also saw many other remarkable advances in the processes of production, preservation and administration in 2010.

THE ENEMY RUNS AWAY BEFORE STRIKE BY VACCINE ARMY

Alarm bells rang around the world in 2009 when the Influenza A H1N1 outbreak was reported. The first laboratory-confirmed cases of H1N1 influenza appeared in Mexico in February and March 2009. It was declared a pandemic by the WHO on 11 June 2009. The illness was caused by a new strain of the influenza virus. The pandemic affected 60.8 million people.[37]

The global response was swift, and vaccine researchers produced vaccines without taking much time. The first vaccine was licenced in August 2010. Indian vaccine manufacturers also worked at lightning speed. The first H1N1 vaccine in India was developed by Cadila Healthcare Ltd and was launched on 4 June 2010. This was followed by the launch of vaccines by the Serum Institute of India (SII), Bharat Biotech and Panacea Biotec.

Fortunately, the pandemic could be controlled. On 10 August 2010, the WHO announced that the H1N1 influenza virus had entered into its post-pandemic period. As many as 18,500 people died of the disease globally, and more than 1,000 people were killed by the virus in India. However, some reports accused the WHO of creating unjustified fears about the health risks faced by people.[37]

Millions of doses of vaccine remained unused, inviting severe criticism of the way in which the WHO handled the outbreak. Although 78 million doses of vaccines were sent by WHO to seven countries, they arrived long after they would have done the most good.[39] Moreover, in Sweden, where more than 60 per cent of the population was vaccinated with the H1N1 vaccine, hundreds of people were later diagnosed with narcolepsy. Millions of others were traumatized.

COVID-19: THE LATEST CHALLENGE TO VACCINOLOGY

The world is now fighting another scourge. A pandemic that is bigger and deadlier than the infamous Spanish flu, COVID-19, is caused by the SARS-CoV-2 virus. It emerged in Wuhan, China, in December 2019 and was declared a pandemic by the WHO on 11 March 2020.

The pandemic has led to numerous research institutes and companies worldwide developing vaccines that target this novel disease. Results came in fast. According to the COVID-19 vaccine tracker developed by the London School of Hygiene and Tropical Medicine (LSHTM), as on 7 March 2022, there were 340 vaccine candidates, of which 112 were in their clinical testing phase; 30 vaccines were in use, 9 in Phase IV clinical trials and 36 in Phase III clinical trials.[40]

Russia was the first to report the development of its COVID-19 vaccine, named Sputnik V, as early as August 2020. The next was Pfizer-BioNTech's COVID-19 vaccine, which received Emergency Use Authorization (EUA) in the USA on 11 December 2020.

India was one of the leaders in COVID-19 vaccine development and production. While the Drug Controller General of India (DCGI) fast-tracked the vaccine licensing process, the Indian Council of Medical Research (ICMR) tied up with a vaccine manufacturer, Bharat Biotec, to develop an indigenous COVID-19 vaccine. Simultaneously, private vaccine manufacturers forged partnerships for the production of vaccines.

Two vaccines were granted emergency use authorization in India on 3 January 2021. These were Covaxin and Covishield. Covaxin was developed by Bharat Biotech in collaboration with the ICMR. It uses an inactivated virus with adjuvants.

An exuberant Indian Prime Minister declared at a meeting of the Chief Ministers of the states on the COVID-19 situation and the rollout of vaccination on 11January 2021: 'It is a matter of pride for all of us that the two vaccines that have been given emergency use authorization are both made in India.'[41] These two vaccines were used to roll out India's COVID-19 vaccination drive from 16 January 2021. But, there were many vaccines in the queue.

On 2 July 2021, India's vaccine regulator, the DCGI, granted a licence to Panacea Biotec to manufacture Sputnik V in India. Biological E was granted permission to manufacture the Janssen

Vaccine on 18 August 2021. This was followed two days later by Cadila Healthcare's approval for the manufacture of ZyCoV-D. On 28 December 2021, two more COVID-19 vaccines, the SII's Covovax and Biological E.'s Corbevax, were added to India's vaccine-manufacturing basket for restricted use in an emergency situation.

There are many other vaccines at different stages of development in India, and the Indian government's mission COVID Suraksha is providing technical and financial support to 30 vaccine candidates.

The strength in vaccine manufacturing that India has demonstrated during COVID-19 is not an overnight wonder. The hard work of Indian scientists, the outstanding entrepreneurship of its business community, its favourable government policies and the availability of manpower have over the years turned India into the 'world's largest vaccine pharmacy'. The next chapter is about how a country that was heavily dependent on the import of vaccines has become the largest vaccine exporter.

REFERENCES

1. Timeline. The history of vaccines [Internet]. History of vaccines.org. 2021 [cited 24 May 2021]. Available from: https://www.historyofvaccines.org/timeline#EVT_100871
2. Pasteur L, Chamberland R. Summary report of the experiments conducted at Pouilly-le-Fort near Melun on the anthrax vaccination, 1881. *The Yale Journal of Biology and Medicine*. 2002 January;75(1):59.
3. Misgie F, Atnaf AA, Surafel K. A review on anthrax and its public health and economic importance. *Acad J Anim Dis*. 2015;4(3):196–204.
4. Timeline. The history of vaccines [Internet]. Historyofvaccines.org. 2021 [cited 24 May 2021]. Available from: https://www.historyofvaccines.org/timeline#EVT_100876
5. Plotkin SA, editor. *History of vaccine development*. Berlin: Springer Science & Business Media; 2011.
6. Louis Pasteur and the development of the attenuated vaccine. VBI Vaccines [Internet]. VBI Vaccines. 2021 [cited 24 May 2021]. Available from: https://www.vbivaccines.com/evlp-platform/louis-pasteur-attenuated-vaccine/
7. Barth R, Gruschkau H, Bijok U, Hilfenhaus J, Hinz J, Milcke L, Moser H, Jaeger O, Ronneberger H, Weinmann E. A new inactivated tissue culture

rabies vaccine for use in man: Evaluation of PCEC vaccine by laboratory tests. *Journal of Biological Standardization*. 1984 January;12(1):29–46.

8. Waldemar Haffkine: The vaccine pioneer the world forgot [Internet]. *BBC News*. 2021 [cited 24 May 2021]. Available from: https://www.bbc.com/news/world-asia-india-55050012
9. Löwy I. From guinea pigs to man: The development of Haffkine's anticholera vaccine. Journal *of the History of Medicine and Allied Sciences*. 1992 July 1;47(3):270–309.
10. Hankin EH. Remarks on Haffkine's method of protective inoculation against cholera. *British Medical Journal*. 1892 September 10;2(1654):569.
11. Nanobot Medical Animation Studio. First plague vaccine: Vladimir Khavkin [Internet]. Nanobot Medical Animation Studio. 2021 [cited 24 May 2021]. Available from: https://nanobotmedical.com/first_plague_vaccine/
12. Chernin E. Ross defends Haffkine: The aftermath of the vaccine. Associated Mulkowal disaster of 1902. *Journal of the History of Medicine and Allied Sciences*. 1991 April 1;46(2):201–218.
13. Hawgood BJ. Waldemar Mordecai Haffkine, CIE (1860–1930): Prophylactic vaccination against cholera and bubonic plague in British India. *Journal of Medical Biography*. 2007 February;15(1):9–19.
14. Kaufmann SH. Remembering Emil von Behring: From tetanus treatment to antibody cooperation with phagocytes. *mBio*. 2017 February;8(1).
15. Linton DS. *Emil von Behring: Infectious disease, immunology, serum therapy*. Philadelphia, PA: American Philosophical Society. 2005.
16. Plotkin SA, Plotkin SL. The development of vaccines: How the past led to the future. *Nature Reviews Microbiology*. 2011 December; 9(12):889–893.
17. Hardy A. Straight back to barbarism: Antityphoid inoculation and the Great War, 1914. *Bulletin of the History of Medicine*. 2000 July 1;74(2):265–290.
18. Osler W. Compulsory anti-typhoid vaccination. *The Times*. 29 August 1914. 29.
19. Gröschel DH, Hornick RB. Who introduced typhoid vaccination: Almroth Wright or Richard Pfeiffer? *Reviews of Infectious Diseases*. 1981 November 1;3(6):1251–1254.
20. Immunology [Internet]. Encyclopedia Britannica. 2021 [cited 24 May 2021]. Available from: https://www.britannica.com/science/history-of-medicine/Immunology
21. Lahariya C. A brief history of vaccines and vaccination in India. *The Indian Journal of Medical Research*. 2014 April;139(4):491.
22. Towey F. Léon Charles Albert Calmette and Jean-Marie Camille Guérin. *The Lancet Respiratory Medicine*. 2015 March 1;3(3):186–187.
23. Luca S, Mihaescu T. History of BCG vaccine. *Maedica*. 2013 March 1;8(1):53–58.
24. Bryder L. 'We shall not find salvation in inoculation': BCG vaccination in Scandinavia, Britain and the USA, 1921–60. *Social Science & Medicine*. 1999; 49(9):1157–1167.

25. Feldberg GD. *Disease and class: Tuberculosis and the shaping of modern North American society*. New Brunswick: Rutgers University Press; 1995.
26. Gomber S, Taneja DK, Mohan K. Awareness of pulse polio immunisation. *The Indian Journal of Pediatrics*. 1996 January;63(1):99–103.
27. WHO South-East Asia region certified polio-free [Internet]. WHO.int. 2021 [cited 24 May 2021]. Available from: https://www.who.int/southeastasia/news/detail/27-03-2014-who-south-east-asia-region-certified-polio-free
28. Stratton KR, Howe CJ, Johnston RB. *Adverse events associated with childhood vaccines: Evidence bearing on causality*. Washington, D. C., WA: National Academy Press; 1994.
29. Hovern D. *The trials and triumphs of the American polio vaccine*. Glassboro, NJ: Rowan University.
30. Weller TH, Robbins FC, Enders JF. Cultivation of poliomyelitis virus in cultures of human foreskin and embryonic tissues. *Proceedings of the Society for Experimental Biology and Medicine*. 1949 October;72(1):153–155.
31. Koprowski H, Jervis GA, Norton TW. Immune responses in human volunteers upon oral administration of a rodent-adapted strain of poliomyelitis virus. *Am J Hyg*. 1952;55:108–126.
32. Salk JE, Krech U, Youngner JS, Bennett BL, Lewis LJ, Bazeley PL. Formaldehyde treatment and safety testing of experimental poliomyelitis vaccines. *American Journal of Public Health and the Nations Health*. 1954 May;44(5):563–570.
33. Blume S, Geesink I. A brief history of polio vaccines. *Science*. 2000;288:1593–1614.
34. Watanabe T, Kawaoka Y. Pathogenesis of the 1918 pandemic influenza virus. *PLoSPathog*. 2011 January;7(1):e1001218.
35. Barberis I, Myles P, Ault SK, Bragazzi NL, Martini M. History and evolution of influenza control through vaccination: from the first monovalent vaccine to universal vaccines. *Journal of Preventive Medicine and Hygiene*. 2016 September;57(3):E115.
36. Harrison LH. Prospects for vaccine prevention of meningococcal infection. *Clinical Microbiology Reviews*. 2006 January 1;19(1):142–164.
37. Enserink M. WHO declares official end to H1N1 'swine flu' pandemic. *Science Insider*. 2010. Available from: https://www.science.org/content/article/who-declares-official-end-h1n1-swine-flu-pandemic
38. Immunization, vaccines and biologicals [Internet]. Who.int. 2022 [cited 15 January 2022]. Available from: https://www.who.int/teams/immunization-vaccines-and-biologicals/diseases
39. Fineberg HV. Pandemic preparedness and response: lessons from the H1N1 influenza of 2009. *New England Journal of Medicine*. 2014 April 3;370(14):1335–1342.
40. COVID-19 vaccine tracker [Internet]. Vac-lshtm.shinyapps.io. 2021 [cited 24 May 2021]. Available from: https://vac-lshtm.shinyapps.io/ncov_vaccine_landscape/

41. PM's closing remarks at meeting with CMs on Covid 19 situation and vaccination rollout [Internet]. PMO India. 2021 [cited 15 January 2022]. Available from: https://www.pmindia.gov.in/en/news_updates/pms-closing-remarks-at-meeting-with-cms-on-covid-19-situation-and-vaccination-rollout/?comment=disable&tag_term=pmspeech

Chapter 3

India's Vaccine Growth Story: World's Vaccine Pharmacy

India's vaccine industry has been on a roller-coaster ride since the advent of vaccines. Beginning with a heavy dependence on import of vaccines, it graduated to sufficient indigenous production. After a few decades of import, entrepreneurs in the country made themselves not only self-reliant but also produced surplus vaccines for export worldwide. Do you know who was the first vaccine producer in India?

CHILDREN, THE FIRST VACCINE PRODUCERS

The first vaccine in India was produced by a three-year old girl named Anna Dusthall. She was vaccinated with cowpox vaccine, which had arrived from Baghdad, along with 19 other children. While others failed to produce pox blisters, Dusthall did not disappoint.

Fluid was harvested from her pustules, five children were inoculated and the remaining material was filled in vials. The children and the vials were dispatched to different parts of the country.

Initially, the smallpox vaccine was produced by inoculating children. Fluid was extracted from their blisters to vaccinate others. Children often accompanied vaccinators on vaccine-related expeditions.

The process was painful, unethical, unsustainable and prone to the transmission of diseases such as syphilis and hepatitis.

Moreover, the parents often opposed experiments on their children. However, the children continued to shoulder the global vaccine production burden for a century. Finally, the practice of arm-to-arm vaccination was stopped in 1890.

Who produced vaccines after that?

ROLE OF COWS, BUFFALOES AND GOATS AS VACCINE PRODUCERS

Slowly, cows replaced children as vaccine producers. The process was the same. The animals were injected with cowpox or smallpox matter; fluid was collected from the resultant pustules and used to inoculate people.[1]

Bombay Presidency took the lead. In 1869, Dr Henri Jules Blanc, Deputy Surgeon in the Bombay Medical Department, brought back vaccines from Belgium and trained local people to inoculate calves. Madras Presidency adopted the process 10 years later.[2]

In view of the Hindus' religious sentiments towards cows, other animals such as buffaloes, goats and donkeys were also used for the production of the smallpox vaccine. Inoculated animals from depots were taken on vaccine-related trips to villages. Excess fluid from pustules was collected in capillary tubes and sent to distant places for vaccination purposes.

Later, institutes for smallpox vaccine production from animals were set up in each province.[3] However, till 1850, the production was insufficient to cater to the demand, which led to imports.

Vaccines would lose their potency in hot weather. Therefore, research started on preserving the quality of vaccines.[3] The first preservative, glycerine, was discovered in 1895. Other additives such as lanoline, vaseline and boric acid were also tried.[2]

As the world got a better grip on the smallpox 'demon', scientists focused on other pathogens. But, the arsenal had to be produced differently.

PUBLIC INSTITUTES USHER IN THE ERA OF LAB-GROWN VACCINES

The British rulers of India were concerned about the mounting deaths of their personnel from tropical diseases. The main scourges were plague, leprosy, cholera and malaria.[3] Moreover, sending soldiers bitten by rabid dogs for treatment to the Pasteur Institute in Paris was burdening the exchequer. Therefore, they decided to set up a series of bacteriological laboratories and Pasteur Institutes across India.[4]

It began in 1881 when the British equipped a small laboratory in Calcutta for cholera research.[5] A bacteriological laboratory was established at Kasauli in 1884 and Agra in 1892.[1,4] The first Pasteur Institute in India was established in Kasauli in 1900. Subsequently, Pasteur institutes came up at Coonoor, Shillong and Rangoon.

Production techniques were simple. Pathogens are attenuated by heating, passing through animals or mixing with other materials. And although there was a compromise on their safety and standardization, the vaccines were successful in reducing mortality.

By 1930, there were 15 vaccine institutes in India.[6] Let's acquaint ourselves with some of these organizations.

GOVERNOR'S HOUSE BECOMES FIRST VACCINE INSTITUTE

In 1896, when the plague epidemic broke out in Bombay and Poona, the Governor of Bombay requested Dr W. M. Haffkine to develop a vaccine. He was provided two rooms in the campus of the J. J. Group of Hospitals to set up a laboratory. One clerk and three peons were lent to him by the Bombay municipality.

Once the vaccine was tested successfully, more space was needed for its production. Lord Sandhurst, the Governor of Bombay, offered Haffkine a mansion, which had been the Governor's house until a few years ago. This became the Plague Research Laboratory on

10 August 1899. Later, it started production of the cholera vaccine and was named the Bombay Bacteriological Laboratory in 1905. In 1925, it was renamed the Haffkine Institute. In due course, the institute started production of DPT and rabies vaccines as well as OPV and anti-tetanus and anti-snake venom serum.[7] It became one of the public sector institutes selected by the Government of India for technology transfer to produce COVID-19 vaccine when the pandemic engulfed the world in 2020.

LADY LILY'S DEATH LEADS TO ESTABLISHMENT OF MANY INSTITUTES

In 1902, an English lady called Lily Pakenham Walsh died of rabies. She could not get anti-rabies treatment in time. Moved by her death, an American philanthropist, Henry Phipps, donated ₹50 lakh to the Viceroy of India to develop medical institutions. Of this amount, ₹1 lakh was allocated for setting up the Pasteur Institute of Southern India at Coonoor. The institute started functioning on 6 April 1907. It manufactured neural tissue anti-rabies vaccines. Subsequently, it developed and produced the influenza vaccine in 1957, and the trivalent OPV and BPL inactivated rabies vaccine in 1970. Its next product was a vero-cell DNA vaccine for rabies (vero in Latin means 'real' or 'true'). In 1977, the institute was renamed the Pasteur Institute of India.[8]

FIRST CENTRAL INSTITUTE ON THE FOOTHILLS OF THE HIMALAYAS

India needed a Central Research Institute (CRI) to conduct medical research, manufacture vaccines and act as a national referral centre for public health problems. Kasauli, a small, picturesque town in the foothills of the Himalayas, was selected to set up the institute. (One of the Pasteur Institutes of India had already been set up in this town.) The work started in 1904, and the institute was opened in 1906.[9]

CRI Kasauli started production of the anti snake venom serum in 1906 and also developed a vaccine for typhoid fever. In 1911, it developed a neural tissue anti-rabies vaccine, named the Semple Vaccine, after the institute's first director. This was the most commonly used anti-rabies vaccine in the world until 2000.[10]

The institute also developed an anti-cholera vaccine in 1914. Next, it started producing diphtheria and tetanus anti serums in 1953 and 1954, respectively, followed by the yellow fever vaccine in 1958. The Pasteur Institute of North India was merged with the CRI in 1936.[4,10]

THE METAMORPHOSIS OF A HUT INTO AN INSTITUTE OF PREVENTIVE MEDICINE

On 7 November 1899, Lt Col Walter Gaven King, Sanitary Commissioner of Madras Presidency, started a smallpox vaccine depot in a tiny hut in Guindy.[11] Due to his efforts, the depot was soon upgraded to a research institute.

The institute was named the King Institute of Preventive Medicine (KIPM) to recognize the contribution of Col King and was formally opened in November 1905. In 1919, KIPM manufactured the anti-influenza vaccine on a large scale for the first time in India. It also started production of the cholera, typhoid and paratyphoid vaccines.[12]

In 1969, the Department of Virology was started in KIPM, and was named the National Polio Lab in 1993. KIMP played an important role in smallpox eradication.[11]

BUSINESS INTEREST MOBILIZES PLANTERS TOO SET UP A MEDICAL INSTITUTE

The tea planters of north-east India were worried about their business. Hundreds of their workers were dying of malaria and kala-azar. These tea planters joined hands to form the Assam Medical Research Society and contributed to the setting up of the King Edward VII Memorial Pasteur Institute in the hill city of Shillong.

The institute started functioning in 1917. It mass produced vaccines for rabies, cholera, typhoid, paratyphoid and bacteriophage. In August 1945, the Assam Medical Research Society was dissolved and the institute came under the Assam government and later under the Government of Meghalaya.

However, vaccine production, except for rabies, was stopped in 1996 as per the central government's directive. The anti-rabies vaccine was discontinued in 2005 after the WHO's ban on production of the neural-tissue anti-rabies vaccine. The institute then became a training centre, blood bank and food testing centre.[13]

Indian vaccine institutes saw a golden period in the first half of the 20th century. But what led to their decline later?

VACCINE INSTITUTES BECOME WAR CASUALTIES

Drafting of personnel for the army and diversion of resources in the First World War led to a short period of abeyance in vaccine research in India.[4] However, India continued to do well in vaccine research and development till the 1930s. The institutes met the country's requirements for vaccines and antisera.

The Second World War and the socio-political situation in India led to the complete neglect of the research agenda. Consequently, India started falling behind in vaccine technology.

The pressure to meet production targets, the drying up of financial support, the drafting of researchers for army duties, and the lack of institutional mechanisms to foster research and the interdisciplinary approach slowly made the institutes obsolete.[6,14,15]

MOUNTING FAILURES IN THE PUBLIC SECTOR

Indian vaccine institutes continued to function post-independence, although without any radical transformation. Some new institutes were also established.[16]

The elimination of tuberculosis was high on the Indian government's priority list. Therefore, a BCG vaccine laboratory was set up in Guindy in 1948. It met 100 per cent of the demand for BCG vaccines in the country.

By 1971, there were 19 public-sector vaccine-manufacturing institutes in India. However, they failed to upgrade their technology or augment their production. Consequently, despite the government's stated policy of self-reliance in vaccine technology and self-sufficiency in vaccine production, the demand-supply gap widened, leading to the import of vaccines.[14]

The shortage of indigenous vaccines was aggravated by interruptions or complete stoppages in vaccine supplies to public institutions.

MORIBUND PUBLIC SECTOR VACCINE INSTITUTES: DELIBERATE OR JUST APATHY?

On the advice of Dr Sabin during his visit to the Pasteur Institute of India in Coonoor in 1963, the institute started production of OPV. However, in 1977, the institute was asked to stop production on the ground that one of the batches was reactogenic.[17] No action was taken to rectify the problem, and the institute was asked to produce bacterial vaccines.

Haffkine Biopharmaceutical Ltd (HBPCL) started production of OPV in 1997, but production was discontinued soon after due to an allegation that the OPV supplied was not potent.[18] BCG vaccine production at the King Institute in Guindy was stopped in 2008.

A new public-sector vaccine-manufacturing company, Bharat Immunologicals and Biologicals Corporation Ltd (BIBCOL), was set up by the Department of Biotechnology (DBT) in 1987. A technology transfer agreement was signed with Moscow's Institute of Poliomyelitis and Viral Encephalitis, which envisaged repackaging OPV imported from Russia initially, followed by indigenous production within five years. However, indigenous production started only after a decade.[16] According to the annual report of BIBCOL 2020–2021, OPV remains the only vaccine produced by this institute, and that too at a huge financial loss.

The government took over a loss-making private company called Bengal Immunity Ltd in 1984. The company was revived to supply vaccines to the government. However, it was declared financially unviable within a decade and eventually closed.

DBT set up Indian Vaccine Corporation Ltd in 1989 to boost indigenous production of the measles vaccine. Technology was to be transferred by Institut Mérieux, a public-sector company in France. However, the transfer did not fructify and the company was closed.[19]

The institutes lacked focus on research on vaccines. Their priorities changed to epidemiological investigations, disease monitoring, clinical trials and post-immunization studies. This has been attributed to the availability of funds for these activities from the WHO.[16]

The policies of the WHO or UNICEF, liberalization of the Indian economy in the 1990s, and the emergence of private players pushed public vaccine institutes further on the path to sickness.[19]

The sudden suspension of the licences of three public-sector vaccine manufacturers inflicted a grievous injury on public-sector vaccine manufacturing in India. Why did this happen and why was no corrective action taken?

SUSPENSION OF THE LICENCES OF THREE INSTITUTES

In 2008, there was a huge uproar in India when the Central Drugs Standard Control Organisation (CDSCO), the National

Regulatory Authority (NRA), suspended the licenses of three prominent public sector vaccine manufacturers. This followed an inspection of these institutes by the NRA and the WHO's representatives. The Health Ministry simultaneously announced its plan to set up an 'Integrated Vaccine Complex' at Chengalpattu in Tamil Nadu, the home state of the then Union Health Minister Dr Anbumani Ramadoss.

The three manufacturers were the CRI in Kasauli, the Pasteur Institute of India in Coonoor and the BCG Vaccine Laboratory in Guindy. These units were meeting 85 per cent of the total requirement of vaccines under the national immunization programme.

It was alleged that because of the suspension of CRI Kasauli's licence, which was the sole Indian manufacturer of the Japanese encephalitis and yellow fever vaccines, there was a shortage of these vaccines. The government was also accused of importing Japanese encephalitis vaccines from a non-compliant Chinese company.

People questioned the government's decision to associate with the WHO's representatives during the NRA's inspections. This request was declined by the government in 2001.[20] The government was also accused by the parliamentary standing committee of acting in haste.

Some media reports alleged that the then director of the BCG lab in Coonoor facilitated transfer of valuable resources such as seed viruses, guinea pigs and even well-trained people to a new private company.[21]

The Javid Chowdhury Committee, constituted by the Health Ministry to determine the reasons for the suspension of licences and recommend a road map for their revival, also criticized the government's decision. It held that the decision was 'based on an illegal procedure, a flawed appreciation of the issues, and was against the broad community interest'.[20]

The economic consequences of the decision came to the fore soon. Within two years of the closure, the prices of primary vaccines soared by 50 to 70 per cent. Many states faced a critical shortage of vaccines.[5,22] The suspensions were revoked on 26 February 2010.[23]

But what happened to the Integrated Vaccine Complex at Chengalpattu, which was once a pet project of the Health Ministry?

THE CHENGALPATTU SAGA

Thirteen years later, the sprawling integrated vaccine complex wears a deserted and gloomy look. Although the construction work is complete and the facility has the capacity to produce one billion doses of vaccines annually, it is yet to produce even a single vial.

Unpaid wages, staff shortages and mounting financial losses personify the complex. An attempt by the government to onboard manufacturers to utilize the complex's facilities for the production of vaccines failed to find a suitor.[24]

The decision to set up the complex invited strong criticism as soon as it was announced, since numerous existing vaccine production institutes in the government were languishing.[21] However, despite the criticism, the government went ahead and approved the proposal formally at a cost of ₹594 crore in 2012. The delay in execution increased the cost to ₹904 crores.

Let's now find out how exactly the private sector vaccine industry started flourishing in the midst of numerous public sector vaccine institutes.

BIRTH OF PRIVATE VACCINE MANUFACTURERS

Like in many other private sectors, the foundation of Indian private sector vaccine manufacturing was laid by family-owned enterprises. The first brick was laid by Acharya Prafulla Chandra Ray, who set up Bengal Chemical & Pharmaceutical Works Ltd in 1901. The company performed well for half a century before plunging into losses. Next was Bengal Immunity Ltd, pioneered in 1919 by Capt. Narendranath Dutta.

Post-independence, the first private sector manufacturer to enter the vaccine market was Biological E. Ltd in 1953. The Serum Institute of India (SII) Ltd followed in 1966. Next was Panacea Biotech, which emerged to meet the critical need for filling and packaging of OPVs imported in bulk. Later, many scientist- and engineer-led entrepreneurs made their entry into the vaccine industry.

However, the private sector played second fiddle in primary vaccine development and production till the 1980s.[25] Restrictions on foreign investment and the absence of product patents promoted privately held small companies in the vaccine and pharmaceutical business in India till 1990.[26]

Some of the vaccine giants we see in India today were born out of very interesting incidents. Let's talk about the biggest one.

THE DEATH OF A HORSE LEADS TO THE CREATION OF WORLD'S LARGEST VACCINE MANUFACTURER

The story of the origin of the SII, now the world's largest vaccine manufacturer, goes like this:

In July 1966, Cyrus Poonawalla waited desperately for four days for a vial of anti-snake venom serum. A snake had bitten one of his favourite mares and the vial was to arrive from Bombay, which was about 100 miles away.

Poonawalla was an ardent horse lover and had had a sprawling racehorse breeding farm in Hadapsar, near Pune, since 1946. However, although the serum was available at the Haffkine Institute in Bombay, it needed government approval to be provided to Poonawalla. By the time the precious liquid arrived, the mare was dead.

Poonawalla was dejected. He had been donating some of his retired racehorses to the Haffkine Institute for the production of serums and vaccines. His experience made him decide to make the serum on his own, and he founded the SII that same year. He started producing tetanus and snakebite serums in a corner of his stud farm. Slowly, the venture expanded into vaccine production for childhood diseases.

While talking to me, Adar Poonawallah, the CEO of the SII and son of Mr Cyrus Poonawalla, confirmed that his father supplied horses and mules to the Haffkine Institute in the 1960s and 1970s to produce anti-snake venom serum. 'Thereafter, Dr Cyrus Poonawalla decided to do this himself and go up the value chain. He slowly started making vaccines and anti-tetanus serum from horses', he said.

However, Dr Cyrus Poonawalla faced many challenges in expanding his new venture. Access to capital and the government's policies were the most formidable obstacles. Adar said, 'We began with limited access to capital. We didn't have banks willing to lend money, and the government's policies at that time were very restrictive and would take years for permissions to come'.

Poonawalla's small, part-time venture has now grown into the world's largest vaccine-manufacturing facility. It exports vaccines to 170 countries. Every second child in the world receives the first shot of the vaccination with the SII vaccine.

This phenomenal growth was fuelled by many national and transnational factors, which transformed the vaccine industry in India.

THE 1990S: THE GAME CHANGER

Liberalization of the Indian economy in the 1990s was a blessing for the vaccine industry. The licence quota barriers began to be dismantled and investment flows increased. At the same time, there were heartening developments for the Indian vaccine industry abroad.

Global vaccine giants started shunning primary vaccines in favour of newer, more sophisticated and more expensive money-spinners. Between 1998 and 2001, 10 out of 14 major manufacturers stopped production of traditional vaccines, partially or completely. Eight of these were the main suppliers of vaccines to the UNICEF.[27]

This created a global shortage of primary vaccines. The bulk buyers, the WHO, UNICEF and others, started looking desperately for new suppliers of low-cost paediatric vaccines.

The demand-supply gap widened in India with the suspension of production and the stagnant output of public-sector vaccine institutes. Simultaneously, there was an increase in domestic demand as the country embarked on the Expanded Programme on Immunization (EPI) in 1978. This was later expanded and rechristened the Universal Immunization Programme (UIP) in 1985.[18,28,29]

Indian private players grabbed the big opportunity with both hands. They increased their production, developed vaccines, struck deals with international bodies, and met the large demand. Their price, at less than $1 per dose, was unbelievably low.

Production of low-cost vaccines was facilitated by cheap labour, skilled management and technical personnel, the low cost of clinical trials as well as local equipment and technological advancement and improvement in cold storage facilities.[30]

The government's financial support for vaccine development, rising domestic demand due to people's heightened awareness, the huge increase in the population, the expansion of India's UIP and the rise in the number of privately held companies trying hard to produce vaccines at a low cost became the key drivers of India's vaccine industry.[31]

Initially, private Indian vaccine manufacturers relied on mature technologies, which they licensed from abroad. However, with the new patent regime in place, they started nurturing home-grown innovations and developed new and more complex vaccines.[32]

The Indian vaccine industry followed a very simple, two-pronged approach by developing vaccines for neglected tropical diseases (NTDs) as well as cheaper alternatives to available vaccines.

Riding on the strength of a robust scientific base and manufacturing capabilities, the Indian private sector has entered into innovative partnerships with global funding agencies and foreign research institutes. They also joined hands with domestic scientific institutions. The result was the production of new and complex vaccines. The meningitis-A vaccine, developed by the SII for Sub-Saharan Africa, is one such example.

Another example is the inactivated oral cholera vaccine. The pathogen was modified by the International Vaccine Institute (IVI), tested in the field by the National Institute of Cholera and Enteric Diseases, and manufactured by ShanthaBiotech.[33]

The indigenous rotavirus vaccine is another result of collaborative efforts. A rotavirus vaccine strain, isolated by the All India Institute of Medical Sciences (AIIMS) in New Delhi, was transferred to Bharat Biotech International Ltd and tested in collaboration with the US National Institutes of Health and the US Centre for Disease Control.[34]

Interestingly, it was the Government of India that played the most important role in propelling private vaccine makers to a new growth trajectory.

GOVERNMENT'S CATALYTIC ROLE

Strong government support in the last few decades has been the key driver of the Indian vaccine industry. The government has generated a huge domestic demand for vaccines through the expansion of the UIP and concerted awareness campaigns. Moreover, it has supported the vaccine industry through research, financial support and regulatory facilitation.

In view of rapid technological advancements, the Government of India set up the Department of Biotechnology (DBT) in 1986. The DBT was mandated to promote self-reliance in vaccine production.

It had sponsored vaccine-related research and development projects in the public and private sectors.

The Biotechnology Industry Research Assistance Council (BIRAC) under the DBT funds biotech start-ups, entrepreneurs and companies at all stages of vaccine development.[32] The government has also created repositories and biosafety level-4 facilities to support vaccines from bench to Phase II.

The National Biopharma Mission, an industry-academia collaboration, supports vaccine candidates at different stages of their development, including proof-of-concept, optimization, toxicity studies and clinical trials.[32] The Technology Development Board under the Department of Science and Technology provides funds for the setting up of vaccine-manufacturing facilities. The Biotechnology Industry Partnership Programme is another initiative to support vaccine development.[35]

The Translational Health Science Technology Institute of the DBT provides preclinical- and clinical development-related support and imparts training to enhance clinical trial capacity. The ICMR and the Council for Scientific and Industrial Research (CSIR) are also facilitating this work.

The Small Business Innovation Research Initiative of the DBT and the CSIR supports start-ups who come up with innovative ideas and hedges for risks. Another initiative, the New Millennium Indian Technology Leadership Initiative, encourages and supports the novel projects of academia and industry very early in their development. In addition, the Department of Health Research, the ICMR, the Ministry of Health and Family Welfare and other scientific ministries are also funding advancement in vaccinology.

According to the Government of India's DBT, the government has also entered into many bilateral and multilateral collaboration agreements. The Indo-US Vaccine Action Programme, initiated in July 1987, focuses on vaccine production, quality control and delivery methodology.[6] The Ind-CEPI Programme (Coalition for

Epidemic Preparedness Innovations), approved on 27 March 2019, is another significant initiative. Its objective is to achieve epidemic preparedness through rapid vaccine development.

The ICMR has signed a memorandum of understanding (MoU) with the IVI for collaborative research in vaccinology. The DBT has also inked bilateral collaborations with other countries on advances in vaccinology.[32]

The government's efforts have contributed to the growth of the vaccine industry and resulted in the development of low-cost rotavirus and cholera vaccines. Major strides have also been made in vaccine development for malaria, dengue and HIV.[36–39]

Moreover, to attract global vaccine industry giants to invest in India, the government has amended the foreign direct investment (FDI) policy. It has permitted 100 per cent FDI in industrial parks in the biotechnology and life science sectors.

INDIA'S VACCINOLOGY ERA

The concerted efforts of the government and industry have made India the world's epicentre for vaccine manufacturing. India now meets 62 per cent of the worldwide demand for vaccines. It is the only developing country among the top 10 vaccine exporters and has the largest global manufacturing capacity for the WHO's prequalified vaccine production. About 77 per cent of the vaccines produced in the country are exported to more than 170 countries. India meets 90 per cent of the WHO's demand for measles and 40–70 per cent for the DPT and BCG vaccines.[40,41]

According to the Ministry of Commerce and Industries, the value of vaccines exported from India has increased from ₹3,94.8 million in 1996–1997 to ₹64.916 billion in 2020–2021.[42]

India has the largest number of USFDA-approved manufacturing plants in the world outside the USA. Indian industry meets about 60 per cent of UNICEF's vaccine demand. In the case of the WHO, it meets 65 per cent of its demand for the DPT and BCG vaccines, and 80–90 per cent of the demand for the measles vaccine.[43,44]

Indian vaccines' unique selling proposition (USP) has so far been high volume combined with low costs. According to the world's biggest vaccine maker, Adar Poonawalla, the USP of the Indian vaccine industry is quality, affordability and reliability. While talking to me, he emphasized that 'there is a very large reliance on Indian pharmaceutical drugs and vaccines because of our good quality and affordable prices'.

The Indian industry is now giving tough competition to foreign multinationals in the development and marketing of complex vaccines too.[35] Many Indian vaccine-manufacturing companies have also partnered with international agencies to develop new vaccines for diseases prevalent in developing and least developed countries. International partnerships have opened doors for new technology.

To enhance their presence and meet global demand, Indian companies have started taking over vaccine production units in industrialized countries. They have also entered into joint ventures with international players for the manufacture and marketing of vaccines.

COVID-19 saw an increase in the number of collaborations between Indian and global vaccine makers. For example, the SII collaborated with AstraZeneca to produce one billion doses of the Oxford University vaccine and export it to low and middle-income countries. Johnson & Johnson partnered with Biological E. Limited to manufacture the Janssen COVID-19 vaccine. Dr Reddy's Laboratories collaborated with the Direct Investment Fund (RDIF) in Russia on clinical trials and supply of the Sputnik vaccine.

With its strong vaccine-manufacturing capability and capacity, India is likely to play a critical role in meeting the global demand for COVID-19 vaccines. The Indian vaccine market was projected to grow by a compound annual growth rate (CAGR) of 12.5 per cent from 2020 and touch $108.02 billion by 2027.[45]

The Indian vaccine industry also meets the massive demand of India's UIP and preventive healthcare programmes of state governments. It supplies about 1 billion doses of 12 vaccines.[46]

According to the DBT, India has multiple strengths that allow it to remain an undisputed leader in mass production of vaccines at a low cost. These include a large reservoir of scientific human resources, cost-effective manufacturing capabilities, a dense network of research centres of academic excellence and laboratories, biotechnology parks, incubators and over 3,500 biotech start-ups. A vibrant drug and pharmaceutical industry and the largest number of USFDA-approved manufacturing plants outside the USA further add to India's strength in vaccine manufacturing.

India can accelerate its vaccine industry further by increasing its expenditure on research and development as a percentage of sales by industry, providing a mechanism for mitigating financial risk, creating state-of-the-art research facilities, building a strong research-academia partnership, facilitating the link between research and commercialization and enhancing the quality of Indian products.

In the spring of 2009, a new virus caused the H1N1 pandemic, affected 190 countries across the world. India was the obvious choice for the WHO to support development of vaccines. According to a report published in the *DNA* on 14 August 2009, three Indian vaccine manufacturers, SII, Bharat Biotech and Panacea Biotech, were selected by the WHO to develop the H1N1 vaccine in April 2009.[47]

The Indian vaccine industry responded swiftly and developed three vaccines for the contagion in less than 12 months.[48] It proved itself again and brought out two vaccines in less than 10 months when the COVID-19 pandemic struck in 2020.[49]

The future of the Indian vaccine industry looks promising. According to Adar Poonawalla, the essential ingredients for the industry's growth, such as capital and human talent, are now available. 'The progress of the Indian vaccine industry is directly related to the speed and manner in which permissions and licenses are granted. Innovation is possible, provided a framework is available for single window clearances and swift approvals', he told me.

Vaccines are not only the most potent weapons in the fight against infectious diseases, but they also fill the coffers of their vaccine manufacturers The next chapter will unfold these two interesting aspects of vaccinology.

REFERENCES

1. Mushtaq MU. Public health in British India: A brief account of the history of medical services and disease prevention in colonial India. *Indian Journal of Community Medicine: Official Publication of the Indian Association of Preventive and Social Medicine*. 2009 January;34(1):6.
2. Bhattacharya S, Harrison M, Worboys M. *Fractured states: Smallpox, public health and vaccination policy in British India 1800–1947*. Hyderabad: Orient Blackswan; 2005.
3. Lahariya C. A brief history of vaccines and vaccination in India. *The Indian Journal of Medical Research*. 2014 April;139(4):491.
4. Katoch CD, Mathur SJ, Shah B, Roy M, Kumar V, Arora R, Srivastava VK. India with contributions of Indian Council of Medical Research (ICMR) over last hundred years. *ICMR Bulletin*. 2011 November.
5. Report of the committee dated 5 March 1928 on the Organization of Medical Research under the. Government of India, constituted under Mr Walter M. Fletcher. Available from: https://dspace.gipe.ac.in/xmlui/bitstream/handle/10973/40184/GIPE-008578-01.pdf?sequence=3&isAllowed=y
6. Madhavi Y. Transnational factors and national linkages: Indian experience in human vaccines. *Asian Biotech Dev Rev*. 2007;9:1–43.
7. Haffkine Institute. History [Internet]. Haffkineinstitute.org. 2022 [cited 20 January 2022]. Available from: http://www.haffkineinstitute.org/instiprofile.htm
8. Pasteur Institute of India, Coonoor, Nilgiris. [accessed on 30 May 2012]. Available from: http://www.pasteurinstituteindia.com

9. Government of India. *The Imperial Gazetteer of India*. Vol. IV Administrative. New ed., published under the authority of His Majesty's Secretary of State for India in Council. Oxford: Clarendon Press; 1909. 457–480.
10. Milestones of C. R. I., Kasauli [Internet]. Crikasauli.nic.in. 2022 [cited 20 January 2022]. Available from: https://crikasauli.nic.in/Milestones
11. Parthasarathy A. King's prescription [Internet]. *The Hindu*. 2013 [cited 20 January 2022]. Available from: https://www.thehindu.com/features/friday-review/history-and-culture/kings-prescription/article4550980.ece
12. Raman R, A Raman. The pioneers of the King Institute [Internet]. Madrasmusings.com. 2015 [cited 20 January 2022]. Available from: http://www.madrasmusings.com/vol-25-no-9/the-pioneers-of-the-king-institute/
13. Main objectives and responsibilities of the Pasteur Institute, Shillong [Internet]. Megrti.gov.in. 2022 [cited 20 January 2022]. Available from: http://megrti.gov.in/19/04_2.pdf
14. Madhavi Y. Vaccine research: A case for national innovation strategy. *Curr Sci*. 1997;73:25–30.
15. Vashishtha VM, Kumar P. 50 years of immunization in India: Progress and future. *Indian Pediatrics*. 2013 January ;50(1):111–118.
16. Madhavi Y. Vaccine policy in India. *PLoS Medicine*. 2005 May 2;2(5):e127.
17. Madhavi Y. The issue of equity in primary vaccine technology development and its implications on the implementation of vaccine policy in India. *Social Sciences and Health News Letter*. 2001;2:5–17.
18. Madhavi Y. Research and production in the Haffkine Institute: A century and beyond. Association for Consumers Action on Safety and Health (ACASH) News 14. 2000: 13–15.
19. Ramachandran R. Vaccine project: In need of a booster. *The Economic Times*. 1995 July 6. Delhi. p. 10.
20. Ministry of Health and Family Welfare. *Chaudhary committee report*. Government of India. Available from: http://www.mfcindia.org/main/bgpapers/bgpapers2011/am/bgpap2011s.pdf
21. Madhavi Y. Vaccine PSUs: Chronicle of an attenuation wilfully caused. *Vaccine*. 2008 June.
22. Thirty-eighth report on major issues concerning the three vaccine-producing PSUs, namely, the Central Research Institute (CRI), Kasauli, the Pasteur Institute of India (PII), Coonoor. the BCG Vaccine Laboratory (BCGVL), Chennai [Internet]. Hsrii.org. 2009 [cited 20 January 2022]. Available from: http://hsrii.org/wp-content/uploads/2014/04/38th20Committee20Report20-20HFW.pdf
23. Alexander J. Vaccine prices stabilise after PSUs back in production, but after immunisation deaths rise [Internet]. Pharmabiz.com. 2015 [cited 20 January 2022]. Available from: http://www.pharmabiz.com/PrintArticle.aspx?aid=65007&sid=1
24. Shortlisting vaccine/pharmaceutical manufacturers for use of HBL's facilities at Integrated Vaccines Complex (IVC), Chengalpattu, on 'as is where is

basis' for production of Covid-19 and other vaccines 2021 Available from: http://www.lifecarehll.com/tender/view/reference/210b7ec74fc9cec6fb838 8dbbdaf23f7jYODeQ

25. Tandon T. Collective L. Drug Policy in India. IDPC briefing paper, February 2015.
26. The Conversation: In-depth analysis, research, news and ideas from leading academics and researchers. [Internet]. The Conversation. 2022 [cited 20 January 2022]. Available from: https://theconversation.com /
27. Madhavi Y. New combination vaccines: Backdoor entry into India's universal immunization programme? *Current Science*. 2006 June 10;90(11):1465–1469.
28. Ministry of Health and Family Welfare, Government of India. Minutes of the meeting of the National Technical Advisory Group on Immunization. June 2014. Available from: https://mohfw.gov.in/sites/default/files/34683728331418118740.pdf
29. Ministry of Health and Family Welfare, Government of India. Minutes of the meeting of the National Technical Advisory Group on Immunization. December 2016. Available from: https://mohfw.gov.in/sites/default/files/48798238911486636162.pdf
30. IMARC. Indian vaccine market report and forecast 2020–2025 [Internet]. Imarcgroup.com. 2017 [cited 20 January 2022]. Available from: https://www.imarcgroup.com/indian-vaccine-market#:~:text=According%20to%20a%20new%20report,INR%2094%20Billion%20in%202019.&text=Moreover%2C%20with%20advancement%20in%20technology,facilities%20have%20also%20been%20improved.
31. Indian vaccine market report and forecast 2022–2027 [Internet]. Expertmarketresearch.com. 2021 [cited 20 January 2022]. Available from: https://www.expertmarketresearch.com/reports/indian-vaccine-market
32. Swarup R, Sharma A, Logani JM. Building a robust ecosystem for vaccine research in India. *International Journal of Infectious Diseases*. 2019 July 1;84:S7–9.
33. Sur D, Lopez AL, Kanungo S, Paisley A, Manna B, Ali M, et al. Efficacy and safety of a modified killed whole-cell oral cholera vaccine in India: an interim analysis of a cluster-randomised, double-blind, placebo-controlled trial. *Lancet*. 2009 November;374 (9702)):1694–1702.
34. Glass RI, Bhan MK, Ray P, Bahl R, Parashar UD, Greenberg H, et al. Development of candidate rotavirus vaccines derived from neonatal strains in India. *J Infect Dis*. 2005 September;192 (Suppl. 1)):S30–35.
35. Gupta SS, Nair GB, Arora NK, Ganguly NK. Vaccine development and deployment: opportunities and challenges in India. *Vaccine*. 2013 April 18;31:B43–53.
36. McSweegan E. A quarter-century of Indo-US vaccine research collaborations. *Microbe*. 2012;7:561–565.
37. Bhandari NT, Rongsen-Chandola T, Bavdekar A, John J, Antony K, Taneja S, et al. Efficacy of a monovalent human bovine (116E) rotavirus vaccine in

Indian infants: A randomized double blind placebo controlled trial. *Lancet.* 2014;383: 2136–2143.
38. Chauhan VS. Development and licensing of first ever vaccine against malaria. *Indian J Med Res.* 2015;142:637–639.
39. Swaminathan S, Khanna N. Dengue vaccine development: global and Indian scenarios. *Int J Infect Dis.* 2019;84:S80–S86.
40. Pharma industry in India: Invest in Indian pharma sector [Internet]. Investindia.gov.in. 2022 [cited 20 January 2022]. Available from: https://www.investindia.gov.in/sector/pharmaceuticals
41. IVMA Team. The Indian vaccine industry: A brief overview. Indian Vaccine Manufacturers Association (IVMA) [Internet]. Ivma.in. 2020 [cited 20 January 2022]. Available from: http://ivma.in/the-indian-vaccine-industry-a-brief-overview/
42. Export Import Data Bank [Internet]. Tradestat.commerce.gov.in. 2022 [cited 15 January 2022]. Available from: https://tradestat.commerce.gov.in/eidb/ecomq.asp
43. Pricewaterhouse Coopers. *Global pharma looks to India: Prospects for growth.* Pricewaterhouse Coopers; 2010. Available from: https://www.pwc.com/gx/en/pharma-life-sciences/pdf/global-pharma-looks-to-india.pdf
44. Horner R. The world needs pharmaceuticals from China and India to beat coronavirus [Internet]. The Conversation. 2020 [cited 20 January 2022]. Available from: https://theconversation.com/the-world-needs-pharmaceuticals-from-china-and-india-to-beat-coronavirus-138388
45. Fortune. Vaccine market size, share, growth. *Global Industry Report* [2027; Internet]. Fortunebusinessinsights.com. 2020 [cited 15 January 2022]. Available from: https://www.fortunebusinessinsights.com/industry-reports/vaccines-market-101769
46. Top 10 manufactures in vaccine market [Internet]. Meticulousblog.org. 2022 [cited 20 January 2022]. Available from: https://meticulousblog.org/top-10-companies-in-vaccines-market/
47. Avian flu takes backseat as WHO wants work on swine flu vaccine first [Internet]. DNA. 2009 [cited 15 January 2022]. Available from: https://www.seruminstitute.com/news_21.php
48. Goel MK, Goel M, Khanna P, Mittal K. Pandemic influenza A (H1N1) 2009 vaccine: an update. *Indian J Med Microbiol.* 2011;29:13–18.
49. Wilson P, Rao A. India's role in global health R&D [Internet]. R4d.org. 2012 [cited 20 January 2022]. Available from: https://www.r4d.org/wp-content/uploads/R4D-Indias-Role-in-Global-Health-RD-Final.pdf

Chapter 4

Vaccine Economy: Lifesaver and Money Machine

Vaccines are a cost-effective and potent weapon for preventing infectious diseases. While they save millions of lives annually, they are also strong engines of economic growth.

SAVIOUR OF MANKIND

'It is within the power of man to eradicate infection from the earth.'

These are the words of Louis Pasteur, who does not need an introduction. The eradication of the dreaded smallpox and the near-extinction of polio from the world have testified these words. Vaccines prevent deadly and debilitating infectious diseases.[1,2] After being administered vaccines, human beings can ward off the attacks of more than 30 pathogens.[3] According to the International Task Force for Disease Eradication (ITFDE), vaccines can eradicate or eliminate many diseases from the planet, including measles, mumps, guinea worm, lymphatic filariasis, cysticercosis and rubella.[3]

Vaccines reached 86 per cent, or 135 million, of the world's infants by April 2019.[1,4] Multiple new vaccines are now being developed at breakneck speed.[1,5]

After a two-decade-long global eradication campaign, the World Health Assembly declared the world free from smallpox on 8 May

1980. In the 20th century alone, this disease claimed around 500 million human lives. Countless more were disfigured and disabled.[6]

India was the favourite destination of this monster.[7] In India, eradication of the disease has saved more than a million lives and prevented many more people from getting disfigured or blinded annually.[7]

In many cases, polio led to irreversible paralysis of various body parts and ultimately to death by immobilizing the patient's breathing muscles. In its peak year, 1981, the number of paralytic polio cases exceeded 450,000.[3]

The Global Polio Eradication Initiative (GPEI) was launched in 1988 to fight the virus through a global vaccination campaign. It led to a sharp decline in polio cases (to just 33) in 2018.[8] Only Pakistan and Afghanistan have the poliovirus circulating even now. Two of the three serotypes of polio have been eradicated.[1,9,10]

It has been estimated that eradication of polio from India has averted 3.94 million paralytic polio cases, 393,918 polio deaths and 1.48 billion disability-adjusted life years (DALYs).[11] India has also eradicated neonatal tetanus.

It has been estimated that the WHO's Expanded Programme on Immunization, launched in 1974, has saved millions of children.[12] Child mortality from diseases for which vaccines are available has come down from 5.1 million in 1990 to 1.8 million in 2017.[13,14] Except for safe drinking water, nothing else has had such a huge impact on reducing mortality in mankind.

The Universal Immunization Program (UIP) has paid rich dividends to India by reducing under-five mortality. Under the programme, the Government of India is providing vaccinations free of cost against 12 vaccine preventable diseases.

According to the Sample Registration Survey published by the Registrar General of India in October 2021, the infant mortality rate in India has come down from 60 per 1,000 live births in 2005 to 30 per 1,000 live births in 2019.[15] Under-five mortality has decreased from 77 per 1,000 live births in 2005 to 39 per 1,000 live births in 2016. The number of deaths of children less than five years of age in India has reduced from 3.4 million in 1990 to 824,000 in 2019.[16]

SOME CHINKS IN THE VACCINE ARMOUR

According to *The Immunization Agenda 2030: A Global Strategy to Leave No One Behind*, prepared by the WHO and endorsed by the World Health Assembly, around 20 million of the world's infants miss out on basic vaccines annually.[1,17] More than 60 per cent of this number is concentrated in just 10 countries, including India; 13 million of the children worldwide do not receive a single vaccine and are considered 'zero-dose' children.[1]

Diseases that are preventable by vaccines claim more than three million lives every year.[18] Diarrhoeal diseases alone claim the lives of more than 500,000 under-five children annually.[4,19]

According to the data, statistics and graphics published by the WHO, despite its more than four-decade-old national immunization programme, only 65 per cent of children in India are fully immunized in time.[20] About one million children in the country still die of vaccine-preventable diseases every year. India accounts for 44 per cent of global under-five deaths from measles, 60 per cent of global diphtheria cases, 44 per cent of cases of Japanese encephalitis, 40 per cent of tetanus cases and 18 per cent of pertussis cases.[21]

BEYOND SURVIVAL: LETTING CHILDHOOD FLOURISH

Vaccines are not only vital for prevention of diseases, but are critical for the development of children. Infectious diseases can lead to reduced school attendance, impaired cognitive development, decreased educational attainment, physical disability and consequently, adult earnings.[22]

Research studies reveal that pneumococcal pneumonia impedes the cognitive development and learning of children and keeps them out of school.[23] Hib Meningitis caused by *haemophilus influenzae* can result in permanent disabilities such as deafness, blindness, paralysis, seizures and intellectual disabilities in 15–35 per cent of survivors.[24] They impair a child's capability to attend school and learn.[25] Measles may lead to blindness; mumps may result in loss of hearing, and intrauterine rubella may lead to cognitive diminution.[23]

Vaccines help to shield children from the impact of infectious diseases on development of their cognitive skills, physical strength and performance at school.[26] Studies have found that children who have been fully immunized with the traditional EPI vaccines were found to have higher cognition capabilities, as measured by their language, mathematics and intelligence test scores, compared to children who did not receive these vaccines.[27]

Children empowered with the *suraksha kavach* (protective shield) of vaccines tend to have more years of schooling and have better educational attainment than those who have not.[1,19] Vaccination in childhood also results in high earnings as adults.[27] Such children contribute more to national prosperity and development than those who have not been vaccinated in their childhood.[1,19]

RETURNS ON INVESTMENT

Investment in vaccines offers a range of economic and social benefits.[19,28,29] The findings from a spate of studies reveal that apart from saving on direct treatment costs, vaccines pay back individuals, families and societies through the improved cognitive development of children, as well as their high educational attainment and skill development, increased lifetime productivity, enhanced income, high consumption, a reduced burden on health systems and absence from work on account of convalescence, and their ability to care for sick people in their families. In addition, vaccines prevent disability, increase savings and lead to higher investment and GDP.[30,31,32]

The benefits of investment in vaccines are harvested repeatedly and over a long period of time. In some cases, the returns accrue over a lifetime. Vaccines promote people's health, which affects economic development through multiple pathways. Healthy children and young adults are more likely to attend and progress through school.[22] They tend to be physically strong and are able to work hard.[22]

The benefits of eradicating diseases by vaccination are huge. It has been estimated that a total investment of $300 million to eradicate smallpox has brought windfall savings of $1 billion every year since 1980.[29,33] Coming to India, the country's total investment in smallpox eradication efforts was $17 million, on which it is reaping benefits of $150 million annually.[34]

Investments of $73 billion in polio eradication efforts have returned $129 billion to governments so far in savings in medical costs alone. Net annual benefits have been estimated at $40–50 billion.[9,35] This has also saved 39.6 million DALYs annually.[36,37] The benefits accruing to India due to polio eradication in the country have been pegged at $1.7 trillion.[11]

Between 2011 and 2020, called the 'Decade of Vaccines', vaccines provided a return of more than 1.5 trillion US dollars.[19] The Decade of Vaccine Economics (DOVE) return on investment analysis in August 2019 estimated in a study of 94 low- and middle-income countries that every $1 invested in measles vaccination provided a return of $76.[5,38] Every US dollar invested led to a return of $24 in the case of DPT and $1.35 in the case of seasonal influenza on health costs alone.[29,31] Increased life expectancy due to vaccines has translated into a 0.3–0.5 per cent increase in annual economic growth.[23]

Studies also show that reduced child mortality and increased life expectancy due to vaccination lead to a reduction in 'replacement births' and 'insurance births' and consequently reduce fertility.[34] This results in additional investment by parents in education, nutrition and the health of their children, and a consequent increase in earnings and adult labour productivity.[39] Vaccines prevent diseases and thereby obviate the need for antibiotics and reduce the prevalence of antibiotic-resistant strains.

At the population level, a reduction in fertility rates decreases the number of young dependents relative to the size of the adult labour force. This change in age structure can lead to increased savings, which can be used to invest in physical and human capital and stimulate economic growth.[23]

High rates of vaccination and reduced disease transmission can make a country attractive for domestic and foreign investment. It also makes affordable technology that enhances economic productivity.[40] In addition, a disease-free environment promotes tourism and immigration.

According to *Making Tourism More Sustainable: A Guide for Policy Makers*, published by the United Nations Environment Program and the World Tourism Organization, the tourism sector is particularly vulnerable to diseases.[41]

During the COVID-19 pandemic, the UN World Tourism Organization estimated a fall of $910 billion to $1.2 trillion in export revenues from tourism in the year 2020. This was expected to have a wide economic impact and a 1.5–2.8 per cent reduction in global GDP.[42]

NEW APPROACH: INCREASED ECONOMIC BENEFITS OF VACCINES

Initially, scholars adopted a narrow perspective to estimate the economic benefits of vaccines. They measured only the gains accruing from saving of treatment costs and short-term productivity losses.[22] They ignored the long-term economic benefits of the absence of diseases and disability, and increased productivity. Moreover, earlier estimates were confined to the impact of vaccine-preventable diseases on vaccinated persons and people closely related to them and not on large populations.

The latest new frameworks to estimate the economic benefits of vaccines include the complete economic impact of vaccines, both narrow and broad. The new frameworks estimate outcome-related productivity gains, behaviour-related productivity gains and the benefits of community externalities.

OUTCOME-RELATED PRODUCTIVITY GAINS

Vaccines help to prevent the negative sequelae of diseases and lead to the consequent improved physical and mental health of people. It results in increased enrolment and attendance in schools, achievements in higher education and increased lifetime productivity.[22] Disease prevention in adults enhances productivity, reduces absenteeism and contributes to economic growth.[28,31]

The new measurement frameworks take into consideration the impact of vaccines on absenteeism, presenteeism and accumulation of lifelong earnings due to improved health, cognition and higher educational achievements.[30,31]

BEHAVIOUR-RELATED PRODUCTIVITY GAINS

Prevention of diseases, consequent improved health and increased chances of the survival of children leads to behavioural changes in society.[22] This brings about economic benefits because of changes in household choices, which are captured by the new economic frameworks.

Vaccination has a demographic impact as well. The decline in infant and child mortality due to vaccination boosts the confidence of parents in the survival of their children. Therefore, they do not opt for more children as 'insurance offspring'. This leads to reduced fertility rates and, consequently, increased investments by parents in each child, leading to improvement in their education and health. Another favourable side effect is that women's participation in the labour force also rises.[22] This results in populations that can better contribute to economic development.[31,43]

COMMUNITY EXTERNALITIES

The benefits of vaccination even spill over to those who are not vaccinated. The new approach to estimating the economic value of vaccines considers community externalities beyond vaccinated people and their caregivers.[22,31]

This includes the herd immunity developed by vaccination, which provides protection to unvaccinated people as well. Increased vaccination rates can affect macroeconomic performance as well as social and political stability. There are gains in welfare too, because uncertainty about future outcomes is reduced.

Analytical studies reveal that vaccines also have macroeconomic effects on, for instance, household consumption, increased foreign investment due to reduced risk and uncertainty, and enhanced labour supply due to demographic changes.[23,44]

New economic evaluation approaches also consider the ecological impact of vaccines, such as reduced antibiotic usage and antibiotic resistance. Moreover, the benefits of platforms developed for delivery of vaccines by using them for health or social care communications are assessed as well.[31]

PROTECTIVE SHIELD FOR ADULTS

Adult immunization prevents infectious diseases and cancers, reduces healthcare costs and the adverse economic and social sequelae of diseases. However, it is a frequently overlooked part of patient care.[45,46]

Several adult vaccines are now available. They provide protection against critical diseases such as tetanus, HPV, hepatitis, typhoid, Japanese encephalitis, meningococcal disease, pneumococcal disease and influenza.

It has been estimated that hepatitis B infected 257 million people in 2015 and claimed 887,000 lives worldwide. The death toll due to the disease continues. This could be prevented by the hepatitis B vaccine, which is 98 per cent effective in prevention of infection and the development of chronic disease and liver cancer. Furthermore, it has been estimated that vaccination can prevent about 50 per cent of deaths from pneumococcal disease and 80 per cent of deaths from influenza-related complications in the elderly.[47]

HPV is the most common reproductive tract viral infection that can cause cervical cancer in women. About one lakh women are diagnosed with cervical cancer every year and 60 per cent of them die from this disease.[46,48] Behavioural changes have been observed in households in which a member has cervical cancer. These changes have a negative impact on educational attainment and earnings.[49]

Research has divulged that inoculation of HPV vaccine has reduced the prevalence of HPV by 83 per cent in girls of 13–19 years of age.[50] It has averted at least 300,000 deaths till 2020.[19,51]

The tetanus vaccine has helped eliminate maternal and neonatal tetanus in 75 per cent of countries. This has had a significant impact on neonatal mortality.[1] However, maternal and neonatal tetanus is still a public health problem in 12 countries in Africa and Asia.

There is now growing attention to 'life-course immunization, which focuses on extension of vaccination from birth through childhood, adolescence, adulthood and into older age'.[52] This includes catch-up vaccinations for the unimmunized and booster doses to address waning immunity.[52]

Adult vaccines can save a lot of money for healthcare systems and families, and reduce morbidity and mortality. However, adult vaccines are yet to gain acceptance and popularity. Before COVID-19, there was only one nationally recommended adult vaccine in India, TT, during pregnancy for the protection of new born against tetanus.

FREEING PEOPLE FROM THE CLUTCH OF POVERTY

Vaccines also provide financial protection to people. In many countries, including India, there are substantial out-of-pocket expenses on healthcare. With the majority of people having limited savings, expenditure on healthcare drags down households into poverty.[1] It has been estimated that up to 63 million people in India are pushed into poverty by health expenses every year.[46]

Vaccines not only prevent infection in the persons vaccinated, but also reduce the risk of transmission of diseases. Reduced infection rates prevent families from getting plunged into poverty by preventing illness and consequent outpatient department visits and hospitalization.[1]

Vaccines also play a critical role in eliminating poverty by preventing losses on account of death and disability and by increasing productivity.[53]

ARE VACCINES MONEY SPINNERS?

For a very long time, the vaccine segment was regarded as a non-profit sector within the pharmaceutical industry. This was because of the expectation of reasonable pricing to enable countries to stockpile vaccines and undertake free vaccination programmes. Consequently, until the early 1990s, many pharmaceutical companies abandoned the vaccine domain.[54]

However, the big companies have slowly started changing the landscape of the global vaccine industry. They expanded into the commercial vaccine market where prices are market-driven, invested in research and development (R&D) for profitable premium vaccines, and adopted new breakthrough technologies to expand their competitive edge and profit potential.[55]

The market also moved towards combating chronic diseases, curing more adults, and using multivalent vaccines. An increased focus on disease-causing organisms with intensive studies on human immunity has opened doors for the advancement of vaccines against non-communicable diseases and cancers. Therefore, after years of neglect, big pharma rediscovered vaccines as a major growth opportunity and not a 'not-for-profit' domain.

The global vaccine market was $33 billion in 2019. High-income countries (HICs) in Europe and the USA accounted for 68 per cent of the total market value.[56] The global demand for vaccines was estimated at 3.5 billion doses in 2018—25 per cent higher than the demand in 2017.[56]

VACCINATION AFFECTING THE STOCK MARKET

The onslaught of pandemics and news of the development of vaccines to combat them has had a huge impact on stock markets globally. When COVID-19 struck and analysts started painting a dire picture of the pandemic, stock markets plummeted across the world in February 2020.[57]

Generally, the stocks of pharma companies, including vaccine makers, gain during pandemics. Riding on the spike in the demand for critical supplies, their profits surge, leading to a beeline of investors.[58] Before COVID-19, the H1N1 pandemic also witnessed a jump in the stocks of Indian drug companies making generic versions of anti-influenza drugs.[59] When Novavax reported encouraging results in its experimental H1N1 vaccine clinical trial in Mexico, its share price turned bullish.[60]

Furthermore, in the fight against COVID-19, as soon as Indian pharma companies garnered attention as potential suppliers of essential drugs, the BSE Healthcare index rose by 36 per cent by the end of 2020.[61] This was a significant rise, considering that overall, the market had gone down by 23 per cent in 2020. NIFTY's pharma index also reported a significant spike during this period.[61,62]

Stock prices have been super-sensitive to any news about vaccines, drugs or the emergence of new variants. As soon as Pfizer and BioNTech announced that their COVID-19 vaccine was 90 per cent effective in trials, global markets surged to record highs.[63] Since beginning of 2020, the shares of major COVID-19 vaccine makers rose continuously. By June 2021, Moderna's shares were up by 850 per cent, BioNTech by 510 per cent and Novavax by 3,620 per cent.[64]

According to the People's Vaccine Alliance, at least nine people associated with vaccine manufacturing were added to the list of new billionaires earning excessive profits from manufacture of COVID-19 vaccines.[65]

However, share prices are volatile and face wide fluctuations due to policy-related announcements and other factors. For example, the shares of US COVID-19 vaccine makers plummeted after the US backed the Indian proposal at the World Trade Organization (WTO) to waive intellectual property protection for the vaccines and other lifesaving products.[66] Evolution of new 'variants of concerns' of Severe Acute Respiratory Syndrome Coronavirus 2 (SARS-CoV-2) led to a dampening effect on the stock market.[67] Just a statement made by the CEO of a vaccine company that its vaccine might not be very effective against the Omicron variant caused a panic in stock markets.[68] But the stocks of major vaccine makers got a boost.[69]

THE VACCINE OLIGOPOLY

The importance of safety and biologics brings strong regulations to the vaccine industry. Development of vaccines is exceedingly capital-intensive, involves highly knowledge-based processes and is risky. The failure rate is high and less than one in ten vaccine candidates achieve licensure. Thus, the entry barriers in the industry are high and difficult to crack for new entrants. Furthermore, investment required for development of new vaccines, large-scale clinical trials to prove the safety of vaccines, scaling up of production and acquisition of technology, leading to acquisition of local producers by bigger players, further limited the competition. This has made the vaccine market oligopolistic.[54,70]

Four large manufacturers, GlaxoSmithKline plc., Pfizer Inc., Merck KGaA and Sanofi, account for 90 per cent of the global vaccine market by value.[70] In terms of volume, the SII Pvt. Ltd, Bharat Biotech, Sanofi and GlaxoSmithKline produce 60 per cent of the vaccines.[70]

Some specific vaccine markets have only one supplier and are thus true monopolies. Thirty-six vaccines have only one or two prequalified suppliers. Nineteen vaccines have three suppliers.[56] The vaccine oligopoly benefits big manufacturers, of which we have only one in India in terms of volume and none in terms of value. Therefore, Indian vaccine makers are not in a position to drive vaccine prices. However, these barriers are slowly being dismantled. How?

BREAKING THE BARRIERS

In the last few years, the high barriers in the vaccine industry have started collapsing. The reverse vaccinology technique, which uses genomic information for vaccine development without culturing microorganisms, has transformed the vaccine-development process. It has reduced the need for intensive tests in animal models that were costly and labour-intensive.[54]

There is a revival of interest in vaccine research and development in the scientific community. Convergence with other streams of science for research and innovative vaccine designs such as proteomics, genomics, immunomics and vaccinology is on the rise. At the same time, government support for vaccine development and immunization has also increased.[71] This has opened the doors of the vaccine industry to smaller players.

Mid-sized vaccine manufacturers, mostly in Asia, have embarked on an expansion path. They are competing in new vaccine markets and regional markets. They offer additional and often more affordable vaccines.[70]

However, the vaccine market is relatively small when compared to the pharmaceutical market. It represents only 2 per cent of all pharmaceutical revenues.

NEW CONTAGIONS AND PANDEMICS TO CONTINUE TO FUEL VACCINE ECONOMY

Due to the emergence of new diseases and pandemics, threats of bioterrorism and the emergence of new technologies, it looks like the vaccine economy is set to see steady growth. Other reasons for the robust growth of the industry in the future include new concepts and multidisciplinary convergence, leading to the development of low-cost, efficacious and safer than before vaccines, and the development of combination vaccines for existing diseases and vaccines for diseases that do not currently have an effective vaccine, for instance, HIV/AIDs, malaria and leishmaniasis.

Expansion in the demand side of the vaccine economy is also likely to push vaccine demand further. Developments in healthcare infrastructure and awareness of the benefits of immunization, a rise in expendable incomes, increased awareness and a rising focus on immunization are some of the key demand-side factors that have a positive impact on the future growth of the vaccine economy.[72]

New methods of administration of vaccines, such as skin patches, aerosols and jet injectors, are being actively developed. The emergence of therapeutic vaccines and vaccines for non-infectious diseases such as addiction, allergies, autism and cancer will further contribute to expansion of the vaccine industry.

According to the Market Research Report published by *Fortune Business Insights*, overall, the global vaccine market is estimated to grow by a CAGR of 10.7 per cent from 2020 to 2027.[73]. From $46.88 billion in 2019, the size of the market is forecasted to reach $104.87 billion in 2027.[73] The growth of the vaccine industry in terms of volume is estimated to be at a CAGR of 6.5 per cent, and from 5.6 billion doses in 2020, it is estimated that the industry will expand to 7.67 billion doses in 2025.[56] The expansion of vaccine markets in India, Brazil and China, where the vaccine uptake rates are still low, will also be a key driver of vaccine growth.[56]

The potential for the evolution and spread of diseases is on the rise today. The risk of outbreaks escalating into epidemics and pandemics is also increasing. This is aided by factors such as population growth, global mobility, urbanization, climate change, increased human-animal contact and shortage of health workers. These factors are expected to spur the growth of the vaccine market in coming years.

Other factors that are expected to drive the vaccine market include strong governmental financial support, competitive pipeline candidates, increased awareness about the importance of vaccination, implementation of national vaccination programmes, rising vaccine coverage and robust R&D for introduction of new products. Adult vaccines are anticipated to have an increased CAGR due to the rise in development of vaccines in this segment. Recombinant, conjugate, subunit and nucleic acid vaccines will be the leading market segments in the near future.[56]

The COVID-19 pandemic has already substantially pushed up the growth of the vaccine industry. This is on account of increasing governmental support for vaccine development and procurement, multiple waves of infection and the growing involvement of international organizations in development of sufficient vaccine facilities.[56] Global coronavirus vaccine revenue was expected to reach $5.75 billion by the end of 2021and the sale in 2022 was pegged at $124 billion.[74,75]

According to the rating agency Care Ratings' report, India's pharmaceutical sector has an opportunity to sell $10 to $11 billion worth of COVID-19 vaccines in the next three years in India and export markets. However, Indian vaccines are likely to fetch a reduced price in the global vaccine market.[76]

The Department of Pharmaceuticals, Government of India, has launched the Production Linked Incentive (PLI) 2.0 scheme. According to Dr Yuvraj, Joint Secretary, Pharmaceuticals, Government of India, the scheme will ensure greater resilience to external shocks, enforce greater drug security and boost the capacity for domestic production of vaccines and high-value products alike. The scheme incentivizes global and domestic players to increase investment and production in the vaccine industry. The PLI scheme is based on the Atmanirbhar Bharat (Self-reliant India) initiative to enhance India's manufacturing capabilities and export in 10 sectors.

INDIAN VACCINE ECONOMY

Currently, vaccines account for about 2 per cent of the Indian domestic pharma market, including consumption under the 'UIP and the private retail market'.[77] 'Although the bulk of the UIP demand is being met by Indian companies, the private market is dominated by multinational manufacturers', said Dr Yuvraj in an interview. Foreign players have a 63 per cent share in the value of the Indian market for high-priced vaccines such as the HPV, pneumococcal, influenza and meningococcal vaccines.

According to the *Indian Vaccine Market Report and Forecast 2020–2025*, the value of the Indian vaccine market in 2020 was Rs 95 billion. It is projected to grow at a CAGR of 18 per cent from 2022 to 2027. The growth of the vaccine market is estimated to be much faster than that of the Indian pharma industry.[78] It is estimated that the market will reach a value of INR 256.5 billion by 2026.[77]

India is the largest producer of WHO-prequalified vaccines. The country is also a major buyer of vaccines. The expansion of the Indian vaccine industry has been attributed to increased public awareness, the government's support for new vaccine development, the increased uptake of the new generation, as well as multivalent vaccines and ready-to-use presentations such as prefilled syringes, needle free delivery.

According to the Government of India's Department of Pharmaceuticals, the Indian vaccine market is split into three verticals, the Domestic Trade Market, Government Business, and the Export Market. According to its value, the export market is about 50 per cent, the domestic trade market around 30 per cent and the government business around 20 per cent.

The domestic trade market in India is dominated by multinational companies such as Pfizer, GlaxoSmithKline and MSD. Indian producers mainly have conventional vaccines in their bags. Despite this, Indian vaccine manufacturers are likely to consolidate their position with the introduction of new products. This is likely to double the current vaccine market to $2 billion in five years [79].

In coming years, big Indian pharma houses are likely to enter the vaccine market because of the high CAGR of the vaccine segment, the eroding margins of pharmaceuticals and the attractiveness of some players in the vaccine business.

Increasing investments by government agencies, the expansion of the UIP, improvement in cold chain storage and vaccine production facilities, technology advancements, the advent of multiple privately owned companies with a focus on innovation and low-cost solutions, rising disposable income, people's increasing awareness, population growth, favourable government regulations, rapid advancements in technology, growing investments, increased advocacy, the acceptability of advanced platforms such as mRNA and a large market for COVID-19 booster doses are also likely to fuel the strong growth of the Indian vaccine market.[79]

'SHIELD' FOR PROTECTION AGAINST ECONOMIC IMPACT OF PANDEMICS

Apart from devastating lives, overwhelming health systems and disrupting delivery of health services, pandemics also result in immense economic losses. Strict public health measures to control a pandemic disrupts normal life and has a huge impact on the economy.[80] Travel, trade, industrial output and overall development is impacted.[1]

The Spanish Flu in 1918 was followed by a recession, and the First World War had a significant role to play in it. The Asian influenza and Hong Kong pandemics also resulted in short economic downturns, although the recovery was fairly quick. However, the stringent response to pandemics in the 21st century has made an increased economic impact.

It was estimated that the SARS pandemic in 2002 led to a $33 cut in global GDP. The major cause of the loss was the impact of the pandemic on tourism in Singapore and Canada.[81] The Ebola outbreak from 2014 to 2016 in West Africa led to an economic and social burden of $53.2 billion.[82]

Economic downturns due to pandemics are clearly visible in the stock market as well. Globally, stock markets nosedived as the COVID-19 pandemic started devastating the world. While announcements of vaccines made a reassuring impact, news of the emergence of variants had a dampening effect on stock markets. This trend was not unique for COVID-19, but was seen in the SARS, H1N1 and Ebola pandemics.

Vaccines are the most potent weapons to contain disease outbreaks and fight pandemics. And they play a powerful role in pushing economies back on the recovery path— more than any fiscal or monetary stimulus.

VACCINE-RELATED RESPONSE TO COVID-19

The economic impact of the COVID-19 pandemic has been particularly brutal. Frequent and long lockdowns to contain the pandemic have led to economic slowdowns around the world.[83] The hardest hit have been the most vulnerable communities.

Jobs were wiped out, essential services were disrupted, and the number of people going hungry increased exponentially. The only way to protect lives, livelihoods and economies and return to life as usual was to roll out an affordable and efficacious vaccine against SARS-CoV-2.[84]

The next chapter is about the unprecedented global efforts, international cooperation and innovations that have led to the development of COVID-19 vaccines at an unprecedented pace.

REFERENCES

1. IA2030 Consortium. Immunization Agenda 2030. A global strategy to leave no one behind. Geneva: World Health Organization; 2019. Available from: https://cdn.who.int/media/docs/default-source/immunization/strategy/ia2030/ia2030-draft-4-wha_b8850379-1fce-4847-bfd1-5d2c9d9e32f8.pdf?sfvrsn=5389656e_69&download=true
2. World Health Organization. Vaccines and diseases. Geneva: World Health Organization; 2019. Available from: https://www.who.int/immunization/diseases/en
3. Plotkin S, Orenstein W, Offit P. *Vaccines*. Philadelphia, PA: Elsevier; 2018.
4. Immunization coverage [Internet]. WHO.int. 2021 [cited 20 January 2022]. Available from: https://www.who.int/en/news-room/fact-sheets/detail/immunization-coverage
5. Strategic Advisory Group of Experts on Immunization. The global vaccine action plan 2011–2020: Review and lessons learned. Geneva: World Health Organisation; 2019 Available from: https://apps.who.int/iris/bitstream/handle/10665/329097/WHO-IVB-19.07-eng.pdf?ua=1
6. Ochmann S, Roser M. Smallpox [Internet]. *Our World in Data*. 2018 [cited 20 January 2022]. Available from: https://ourworldindata.org/smallpox#citation
7. Gelfand HM. A critical examination of the Indian smallpox eradication program. American *Journal of Public Health and the Nations Health*. 1966 October; 56(10):1634–1651.

8. Poliomyelitis [Internet]. WHO.int. 2019 [cited 20 January 2022]. Available from: https://www.who.int/news-room/fact-sheets/detail/poliomyelitis
9. Tebbens RJ, Pallansch MA, Cochi SL, Wassilak SG, Linkins J, Sutter RW, Aylward RB, Thompson KM. Economic analysis of the global polio eradication initiative. *Vaccine*. 2010; December 16;29(2):334–343.
10. GPEI-polio eradication and endgame strategic plan 2013–2018 [Internet]. Polioeradication.org. 2012 [cited 20 January 2022]. Available from: https://polioeradication.org/who-we-are/strategic-plan-2013-2018/
11. Nandi A, Barter DM, Prinja S, John TJ. The estimated health and economic benefits of three decades of polio elimination efforts in India. *Indian Pediatrics*. 2016 August;7:53.
12. LSHTM Vaccine Centre. The power of vaccines [Internet]. LSHTM. 2022 [cited 20 January 2022]. Available from: https://www.lshtm.ac.uk/research/centres/vaccine-centre/about-us
13. Vanderslott S. How is the world doing in its fight against vaccine preventable diseases? [Internet] Our World in Data. 2018 [cited 20 January 2022]. Available from: https://ourworldindata.org/vaccine-preventable-diseases
14. Rhee JH. Towards Vaccine 3.0: New era opened in vaccine research and industry. *Clinical and Experimental Vaccine Research*. 2014 January;3(1):1.
15. SRS Bulletin, Central Registration System [Internet]. Censusindia.gov.in. 2021 [cited 15 January 2022]. Available from: https://censusindia.gov.in/vital_statistics/SRS_Bulletins/SRS%20Bulletin%202019.pdf
16. UNICEF. Levels and trends in child mortality 2020. New York, NY: United Nations Inter-agency Group for Child Mortality Estimation. 2020.
17. History of Smallpox [Internet]. CDC.gov. 2022 [cited 20 January 2022]. Available from: https://www.cdc.gov/smallpox/history/history.html
18. Abubakar II, Tillmann T, Banerjee A. Mortality and causes of death collaborators. Global, regional and national age-sex specific all-cause and cause-specific mortality for 240 causes of death, 1990–2013: A systematic analysis for the Global Burden of Disease Study 2013. *Lancet*. 2015 January 10;385(9963):117–171.
19. Ozawa S, Clark S, Portnoy A, Grewal S, Brenzel L, Walker DG. Return on investment from childhood immunization in low-and middle-income countries, 2011–20. *Health Affairs*. 2016 February 1;35(2):199–207.
20. World Health Organization. Data, statistics and graphics. Available from: https://www.who.int/immunization/monitoring_surveillance/data/en/
21. Megiddo I, Colson AR, Nandi A, Chatterjee S, Prinja S, Khera A, Laxminarayan R. Analysis of the Universal Immunization Programme and introduction of a rotavirus vaccine in India with IndiaSim. Vaccine. 2014 August 11;32:A151–161.
22. Bärnighausen T, Bloom DE, Cafiero ET, O'Brien JC. Economic evaluation of vaccination: capturing the full benefit, with an application to human papillomavirus. *Clinical Microbiology and Infection*. 2012 October;18:70–76. https://doi.org/10.1111/j.1469-0691.2012.03977.x

23. Bärnighausen T, Bloom DE, Cafiero-Fonseca ET, O'Brien JC. Valuing vaccination. *Proceedings of the National Academy of Sciences*. 2014 August 26;111(34):12313–12319.
24. Bärnighausen T, Bloom DE, Canning D, Friedman A, Levine OS, O'Brien J, Privor-Dumm L, Walker D. Rethinking the benefits and costs of childhood vaccination: The example of the Haemophilus influenzae type b vaccine. *Vaccine*. 2011 March 16;29(13): 2371–2380.
25. Chandran A, Herbert H, Misurski D, Santosham M. Long-term sequelae of childhood bacterial meningitis: an underappreciated problem. *The Pediatric Infectious Disease Journal*. 2011 January 1;30(1):3–6.
26. Value of vaccination [Internet]. Gavi.org. 2022 [cited 20 January 2022]. Available from: https://www.gavi.org/vaccineswork/value-vaccination
27. Bloom DE, Canning D, Shenoy ES. The effect of vaccination on children's physical and cognitive development in the Philippines. *Applied Economics*. 2012 July 1;44(21):2777–2783.
28. Postma M, Carroll S, Brandão A. The societal impact of direct and indirect protection from lifespan vaccination. *Journal of Market Access Health Policy*. 2015;3:26962.
29. Bonanni P, Picazo J, Rémy V. The intangible benefits of vaccination: What is the true economic value of vaccination? *J Market Access Health Policy*. 2015;3:26964.
30. Quilici S, Smith R, Signorelli C. Role of vaccination in economic growth. *Journal of Market Access & Health Policy*. 2015 January 1;3(1):27044. Available from: https://doi.org/10.3402/jmahp.v3.27044
31. Vergara F. *The economic impact of vaccination: more than meets the eye*. Available from: https://www.bactivax.eu/blog/the-economic-impact-of-vaccination-more-than-meets-the-eye
32. Sinclair D, Walker T. Immune response. Adult immunisation in the UK. The International Longevity Centre. November 2013.
33. Lessons from 40-year 'victory over smallpox' can be used to combat coronavirus today [Internet]. *UN News*. 2020 [cited 20 January 2022]. Available from: https://news.un.org/en/story/2020/05/1063582
34. Brilliant LB. The management of smallpox eradication in India. Ann Arbor, MI: University of Michigan Press; 1985. Available from: http://www.zero-pox.info/other_docs/brilliant_mgmt_spox_india.pdf
35. Ochmann S, Roser M. *Polio: Our world in data*. 10 October 2017.
36. Khan MM, Ehreth J. Costs and benefits of polio eradication: a long-run global perspective. *Vaccine*. 2003 January 30;21(7-8):702–705. [5.3]
37. Ochmann S, Roser M. *Polio: Our world in data* [Internet]. 2017 [cited 20 January 2022]. Available from: https://ourworldindata.org/polio
38. Johns Hopkins University, International Vaccine Access Center. Methodology report: Decade of vaccines economics (DOVE). Return on investment analysis.

39. Bloom DE, Canning D, Fink G, Finlay JE. Fertility, female labor force participation, and the demographic dividend. *Journal of Economic Growth*. 2009 June;14(2):79–101.
40. Alsan M, Bloom DE, Canning D. The effect of population health on foreign direct investment inflows to low-and middle-income countries. *World Development*. 2006 April 1;34(4):613–630.
41. UNEP. Making tourism more sustainable: A guide for policy makers. United Nations Environment Programme, Division of Technology, Industry and Economics. 2005. Paris. Available from: https://wedocs.unep.org/bitstream/handle/20.500.11822/8741/-Making%20Tourism%20More%20Sustainable_%20A%20Guide%20for%20Policy%20Makers-2005445.pdf?sequence=3&isAllowed=y
42. Tourism and COVID-19: Unprecedented economic impact [Internet]. Unwto.org. 2022 [cited 14 January 2022]. Available from: https://www.unwto.org/tourism-and-covid-19-unprecedented-economic-impacts
43 Sharma R. Health and economic growth: Evidence from dynamic panel data of 143 years. *PloS One*. 2018 October 17;13(10):e0204940.
44. Luyten J, Beutels P. The social value of vaccination programs: beyond cost-effectiveness. *Health Affairs*. 2016 February 1;35(2):212–218.
45. Tan L. Adult vaccination: now is the time to realize an unfulfilled potential. *Human Vaccines & Immunotherapeutics*. 2015 September 2;11(9): 2158–2166.
46. Dash R, Agrawal A, Nagvekar V, Lele J, Di Pasquale A, Kolhapure S, Parikh R. Towards adult vaccination in India: a narrative literature review. *Human Vaccines & Immunotherapeutics*. 2020 April 2;16(4):991–1001.
47. Philippidis A. Top 15 vaccines of 2012 [Internet]. GEN—*Genetic Engineering and Biotechnology News*. 2013 [cited 20 January 2022]. Available from: http://www.genengnews.com/insight-and-intelligenceand153/top-15-vaccines-of-2012/
48. HPV Information Centre. India. Human papillomavirus and related cancers, fact sheet 2018. Available from: http:// hpvcentre.net/statistics/reports/IND_FS.pdf?t=1546505768606
49. Arrossi S, Matos E, Zengarini N, Roth B, Sankaranayananan R, Parkin M. The socio-economic impact of cervical cancer on patients and their families in Argentina, and its influence on radiotherapy compliance. Results from a cross-sectional study. *Gynecologic Oncology*. 2007 May 1;105(2):335–340.
50. Drolet M, Bénard É, Pérez N, Brisson M, Ali H, Boily MC, Baldo V, Brassard P, Brotherton JM, Callander D, Checchi M. Population-level impact and herd effects following the introduction of human papillomavirus vaccination programmes: updated systematic review and meta-analysis. *The Lancet*. 2019 August 10;394(10197): 497–509.
51. Garland SM, Skinner SR, Brotherton JM. Adolescent and young adult HPV vaccination in Australia: achievements and challenges. *Preventive Medicine*. 2011 October 1;53:S29–S35.

52. World Health Organization. *World report on ageing and health*. 2015. Available from: http://www.who.int/ageing/ events/world-report-2015-launch/en/
53. Chang AY, Riumallo-Herl C, Perales NA, Clark S, Clark A, Constenla D, et al. The equity impact vaccines may have on averting deaths and medical impoverishment in developing countries. *Health Affairs (Millwood)*. 2018;37(2):316–324.
54. Rhee JH. Towards Vaccine 3.0: New era opened in vaccine research and industry. *Clinical and Experimental Vaccine Research*. 2014 January 1;(1):1.
55. Greco M. Development and supply of vaccines: an industry perspective. In: Levine M, J B Kaper, R Rappuoli, M A Liu, M F Good, editors. *New generation vaccines*. 4th ed. New York, NY: Marcel Dekker; 2004. 75–87.
56. *Global vaccine market report* [Internet]. WHO.int. 2020 [cited 14 January 2022]. Available from: https://www.who.int/immunization/programmes_systems/procurement/mi4a/platform/module2/2020_Global_Vaccine_Market_Report.pdf?ua=1
57. Patton M. How stocks reacted during past flu pandemics and steps you can take to minimize losses [Internet]. Forbes. 2022 [cited 14 January 2022]. Available from: https://www.forbes.com/sites/mikepatton/2020/02/28/how-stocks-reacted-during-past-flu-pandemics-and-steps-you-can-take-to-minimize-losses/?sh=551e79f2448d
58. Chakraborty C. Market movers: Pharma stocks surge, banks sink; 37 stocks blink sell [Internet]. *The Economic Times*. 2022 [cited 14 January 2022]. Available from: https://economictimes.indiatimes.com/markets/stocks/news/market-movers-pharma-stocks-surge-banks-sink-37-stocks-blink-sell/articleshow/82144865.cms?utm_source=contentofinterest&utm_medium=text&utm_campaign=cppst
59. Reuters. Pharma stocks with swine flu panacea jump [Internet]. *Mint*. 2009 [cited 14 January 2022]. Available from: https://www.livemint.com/Money/4dstrqf7lowZZKpIePSbKM/Pharma-stocks-with-swine-flu-panacea-jump.html
60. Carroll J. Novavax shares surge on promising H1N1 trial data [Internet]. FiercePharma. 2010 [cited 14 January 2022]. Available from: https://www.fiercepharma.com/vaccines/novavax-shares-surge-on-promising-h1n1-trial-data
61. Presswalla R. Pharma sector outperforms in 2020 so far; 4 stocks surge over 50% [Internet]. Moneycontrol. 2020 [cited 14 January 2022]. Available from: https://www.moneycontrol.com/news/business/markets/pharma-sector-outperforms-in-2020-so-far-4-stocks-surge-over-50-5262011.html
62. Mascarenhas F. [Internet]. 2021 [cited 14 January 2022]. Available from: https://www.reuters.com/world/india/indian-shares-rise-pharma-stocks-lead-gains-2021-10-04/
63. Jolly J, Wearden G. Global stock markets surge after Pfizer Covid vaccine news [Internet]. *The Guardian*. 2020 [cited 14 January 2022].

Available from: https://www.theguardian.com/business/2020/nov/09/stock-markets-covid-vaccine-ftse-100-coronavirus
64. Zuckerman G. Vaccine makers face challenge in sustaining winning streak [Internet]. WSJ. 2021 [cited 14 January 2022]. Available from: https://www.wsj.com/articles/stocks-of-covid-19-vaccine-makers-need-a-fresh-push-11622539800
65. Oxfam. COVID vaccines create 9 new billionaires with combined wealth greater than cost of vaccinating world's poorest countries [Internet]. Oxfam International. Oxfam International. 2021 [cited 14 January 2022]. Available from: https://www.oxfam.org/en/press-releases/covid-vaccines-create-9-new-billionaires-combined-wealth-greater-cost-vaccinating
66. Feuer W. Shares of COVID vaccine makers plummet after US backs IP waiver [Internet]. New York Post. 2021 [cited 14 January 2022]. Available from: https://nypost.com/2021/05/06/shares-of-covid-vaccine-makers-fall-after-us-backs-ip-waiver/
67. *Financial Times*. News updates from November 26: Coronavirus variant concerns send global stocks lower, nations restrict travel from southern Africa, Black Friday sales grow as shoppers return to stores [Internet]. Ft.com. 2022 [cited 14 January 2022]. Available from: https://www.ft.com/content/8245c992-4a4d-4110-b10c-b294c41d501c
68. *CBS News*. Stocks slide on Moderna warning about Omicron, Powell comments on inflation [Internet]. Cbsnews.com. 2021 [cited 14 January 2022]. Available from: https://www.cbsnews.com/news/covid-omicron-variant-vaccines-moderna-stock/
69. Monica P. Covid vaccine makers' stocks soar on Omicron variant concerns [Internet]. CNN. 2021 [cited 14 January 2022]. Available from: https://edition.cnn.com/2021/11/29/investing/vaccine-omicron-variant-covid-stocks/index.html
70. ltd R. Vaccines market—Global industry analysis (2017–2020), growth trends and market forecast (2021–2025) [Internet]. Researchandmarkets.com. 2021 [cited 13 June 2021]. Available from: https://www.researchandmarkets.com/reports/5315023/vaccines-market-global-industry-analysis-2017?utm_source=GNOM&utm_medium=PressRelease&utm_code=wlg3tz&utm_campaign=1531451+-+Global+Vaccines+Market+Analysis+Report+2021%3a+Forecast+to+2025+Featuring+Sinopharm%2c+Serum+Institute%2c+Novavax%2c+Moderna%2c+Mitsubishi+Tanabe+Pharma%2c+Emergent+BioSolutions%2c+and+CSL&utm_exec=chdo54prd
71. Bagnoli F, Baudner B, Mishra RP, Bartolini, E, Fiaschi L, Mariotti P, et al. Designing the next generation of vaccines for global public health. *OMICS*. 2011;15:545–566.
72. Vaccines and market—Forecast to 2024 [Internet]. Marketsandmarkets.com. 2022 [cited 20 January 2022]. Available from: https://www.marketsandmarkets.com/Market-Reports/vaccine-technologies-market-1155.html

73. Fortune. Vaccines market size, share, growth: Global industry report [2027; Internet]. Fortunebusinessinsights.com. 2020 [cited 15 January 2022]. Available from: https://www.fortunebusinessinsights.com/industry-reports/vaccines-market-101769
74. Brandessence Market Research And Consulting Private Limited. 'Coronavirus vaccine market size is projected to reach 75.75 billion by the end of 2021', says Brandessence Market Research [Internet]. Prnewswire.com. 2022 [cited 20 January 2022]. Available from: https://www.prnewswire.com/in/news-releases/-corona-virus-vaccine-market-size-is-projected-to-reach-75-75-billion-by-end-of-2021-says-brandessence-market-research--873560019.html
75. Dunleavy K. Pfizer, Moderna will rake in a combined $93 billion next year on COVID-19 vaccine sales: report [Internet]. FiercePharma. 2021 [cited 15 January 2022]. Available from: https://www.fiercepharma.com/pharma/pfizer-moderna-will-rake-a-combined-93-billion-next-year-covid-19-sales-says-analytics-group
76. COVID-19 vaccine: $11 billion global market opportunity for India, says report [Internet]. *The Hindu*. 2021 [cited 14 January 2022]. Available from: https://www.thehindu.com/business/Industry/covid-19-vaccine-11-billion-global-market-opportunity-for-india-says-report/article35951758.ece
77. Imarc. Indian Vaccine Market Report and Forecast 2020–2025 [Internet]. Imarcgroup.com. 2017 [cited 20 January 2022]. Available from: https://www.imarcgroup.com/indian-vaccine-market
78. Vashishtha VM, Kumar P. 50 years of immunization in India: Progress and future. *Indian Pediatrics.* 2013 January 1;50(1):111–118.
79. EMR. Indian vaccine market report and forecast 2022–2027 [Internet]. Expertmarketresearch.com. 2022 [cited 14 January 2022]. Available from: https://www.expertmarketresearch.com/reports/indian-vaccine-market
80. Ip G, Dougherty D, Debarros A. Lessons for the coronavirus crisis from six other disasters. WSJ Newsletter. 2020.
81. Begley S. Flu-conomics: The next pandemic could trigger global recession. Reuters. Available from: https://www.reuters.com/article/us-reutersmagazine-davos-flu-economy/flu-conomics-the-next-pandemic-could-trigger-global-recession-idUSBRE90K0F820130121
82. Huber C, Finelli L, Stevens W. The economic and social burden of the 2014 Ebola outbreak in West *Africa. J Infect Dis.* 2018;218. suppl. 5: S698–704.
83. Jones L, Palumbo D, Brown D. Coronavirus: How the pandemic has changed the world economy. *BBC News.* 24 January 2021.
84. Anyiam-Osigwe T. Is there an economic case for global vaccinations? [Internet]. Gavi.org. 2021 [cited 20 January 2022]. Available from: https://www.gavi.org/vaccineswork/there-economic-case-global-vaccinations#:~:text=In%20this%20more%20optimistic%20scenario,more%20than%20US%24%202%20trillion.

Chapter 5

Developing Vaccines at Pandemic Speed

A NEW CONTAGION STRIKES MANKIND

On the joyful afternoon on 31 December 2019, people were gearing up to welcome the New Year, with intense celebrations. But a handful of people sitting in the WHO's office in the People's Rcpublic of China were anxious. The Wuhan Municipal Health Commission had declared that it had detected a cluster of cases of pneumonia of an unknown nature.[1]

On 7 January 2020, the Chinese authorities finally isolated the causative organism, a novel coronavirus. It was later named the SARS-CoV-2 and the disease was called COVID-19.[2]

Genetic sequencing of the virus was carried out and shared with the world on 12 January 2020.[3] By 20 January 2020, the disease had spread to Thailand, Japan and the Republic of Korea.[4] The WHO declared it a Public Health Emergency of International Concern on 30 January 2020 and a pandemic on 11 March 2020.

Due to its novel nature, the world lacked vaccines and chemotherapeutic interventions against SARS-CoV-2. The highly infectious virus had struck mankind with unprecedented force and created an unparalleled existential crisis.

Initially, countries responded with soft public health measures such as screening, quarantine and social distancing. When these measures could not stem the spread of the disease, sealing of

outbreak hotspots, lockdowns and curfews were resorted to. This impeded economic activity and shattered livelihoods.

By 11 April 2022, the world had seen at least three waves of the disease, with the number of confirmed cases reported to the WHO mounting to 497,057,239 (including 6,179,104 deaths).[5] India reported 4,30,36,928 cases, including 521,710 deaths.[6]

ILLUSIVE SEARCH FOR 'PATIENT ZERO'

The search for the first human infected by the virus, called 'patient zero' or the index case, began as soon as the new virus was reported. This was critical to establishing new zoonotic reservoirs and preventing re-infection.[7] Early cases revealed an association with the Huanan Seafood Wholesale Market in Wuhan, China, and suggested a human-animal interface.

However, retrospective investigations concluded that the first patient of COVID-19 who reported to a hospital on 1 December 2019 had no links with the Huanan market.[7,8,9] Subsequent genome analysis and studies suggested that the virus had jumped from animals to humans as early as September 2019.[7,8,10,11]

Conclusive proof of how and when the contagion crossed over to humans is yet to be unravelled.[8] In spite of innumerable controversial theories on the internet, finding patient zero for COVID-19 remains elusive.[7]

DID THE MONSTER EMERGE NATURALLY?

China is a strong proponent of the theory of the natural origin of SARS-CoV-2. It posited that the contagion emerged simultaneously in different countries.[12,13] Some viral genome experts are of the view that the virus is closely related to a coronavirus that came from a bat in a cave in China in 2014.

On 18 May 2020, the World Health Assembly resolved to identify the zoonotic source of the virus and the route of its introduction to the human population.[14] But due to stiff resistance from China, the joint team could only visit the country in January 2021, and that too, under strict limitations.[15,16]

The team's report, published on 30 March 2021, brought out that SARS-CoV-2 jumping from bats to humans via an intermediary animal was the most probable reason for the spread of the disease. The virus escaping from a laboratory was the least probable of the four scenarios considered.[7] However, the report categorically stated that the data examined was insufficient.[16]

The inclusion of 17 Chinese scientists in the team, the lack of access to complete, original data and samples about the early stages of the outbreak, inability to find the intermediate host and China's refusal to share the activity log of scientists at the Wuhan Lab also affected the credibility of the report.[12,13,17,18,19] According to a section of experts, the conclusions lacked scientific justification and the lab leak hypothesis was given only a cursory look.[20]

Countries including India demanded a comprehensive, independent, expert-led investigation to determine the origin of the pandemic.[12,17,18,20]

DID THE VIRUS ESCAPE FROM A LAB?

As the pandemic ravaged nations, voices proffering scientific evidence in favour of a lab leak grew louder. The Huanan market, the initial epicentre of COVID-19, is just 25–30 kilometres from the Wuhan Institute of Virology (WIV). Scientists at the institute conduct research on coronaviruses, including on the SARS-CoV-2 family.[13]

The inability to identify the intermediary host, lack of total access to the WIV, and adequate mutations in a bat virus to be infective to humans supplemented the lab-leak theory.[17,21] The bat species believed to be the source of SARS-CoV-2 is found around 1,500 kilometres from Wuhan.[13] Therefore, the contagion could not have appeared in Wuhan without infecting people en route.[13]

In a paper, two Chinese researchers, Botao Xiao and Lei Xiao, also claimed that the killer coronavirus originated from the Wuhan lab. However, their conclusions were based on assumptions and lacked scientific evidence. Stating that the bats carrying the SARS-CoV-2 were originally found in the Yunnan or Xhejiang provinces, which were about 900 km from Wuhan, they concluded that the possibility of bats reaching Wuhan was slim.

In May 2021, Republican members of the US House Permanent Select Committee on Intelligence (HPSCI) released a report titled *Covid-19 and the Wuhan Institute of Virology*. The report claimed that 'significant circumstantial evidence' exists for the viral leak from WIV.[22]

According to a US intelligence report, many researchers working at the WIV had to be hospitalized in November 2019, with symptoms consistent with COVID-19.[12,13,23,24] However, the Director of National Intelligence said that both the natural origin and a lab leak are plausible hypotheses for the first infection of a human being by SARS-CoV-2. British intelligence agencies have also agreed about the feasibility of emergence of the pandemic through a viral leak.[25]

According to some reports, the virus found it difficult to adjust back to bats, which suggests that it was genetically engineered in a lab.[13,26] A section of scientists believe that SARS-CoV-2 originated from 'gain of function' research. In such research, pathogens are genetically engineered to make them more infectious. Fingers were pointed at Shi Zhengli, a top Chinese virologist who is also known as the 'Bat Woman of China'.[27,28]

SEARCH FOR A SAFE AND EFFICACIOUS VACCINE

The commitment of huge resources on public health interventions was unable to vanquish the contagion. As the pandemic unfolded, the world increasingly turned to vaccines to save lives and take the global economy on a recovery path. Thus, an unprecedented global quest for COVID-19 vaccines began.[29]

However, development of vaccines is a cost-intensive process, and often spills over a decade. Vaccine-manufacturing also requires highly regulated and expensive facilities. How would the world get a COVID-19 vaccine at such a breakneck speed?

ACCELERATED VACCINE DEVELOPMENT ENDEAVOURS IN THE PRE-COVID-19 ERA

Scientists and manufacturers have experimented with compressed vaccine development timelines during past outbreaks. In the case of the H1N1/Swine-Flu outbreak in 2009, vaccines were developed swiftly.[30] This was made possible by existing, well-developed influenza vaccine technologies and licencing of vaccines under the rules.

In the case of the Ebola outbreak in West Africa in 2014, scientists used an existing technology developed for the HIV vaccine for a swift outcome.[30] Phase 3 trials started within a year of the eruption of the pandemic. Although the vaccine was used on 'compassionate' grounds to control an epidemic in Congo in 2018, it could only be licensed in 2019.

Development of vaccines for the Zika, Severe Acute Respiratory Syndrome (SARS) and Middle East Respiratory Syndrome (MERS) viruses also began at a rapid pace. But none of them went past the first stages of development and testing before the virus disappeared.

DEVELOPING A VACCINE IN A FEW MONTHS

In the case of COVID-19, the global humanitarian crisis created a state of *force majeure*. It challenged the orthodoxy in vaccine development and resulted in churning out of vaccines at a dizzying pace.

The colossal efforts of contagion led governments, scientists and manufacturers to find ways to chop not just months but years off the timeline, led to success. The discovery phase, the lead candidate optimization, the preclinical studies and starting of clinical trials happened within two months of the onset of the pandemic.

A rich bouquet of vaccines was ready in less than a year of declaration of the disease as a Public Health Emergency of International Concern. But how was this monumental feat achieved?

UNPRECEDENTED COLLABORATION

Intense global collaboration will be remembered in history as the reason for the COVID-19 vaccine development. Industry, academia, regulatory bodies, philanthropists and governments joined hands to develop multiple, safe and effective vaccines.

While the USA launched Operation Warp Speed, the Indian government came up with Mission COVID Suraksha. Many other governments and the European Commission have also funded vaccine candidates.

A global collaborative project, the Access to COVID-19 Tools Accelerator (ACT-A), was launched in April 2020 to fight COVID-19. It has four pillars: vaccines, therapeutics, diagnostics and the foundational Health System Connector.

The COVAX facility, the vaccine pillar of the ACT-A, was founded by the WHO, the GAVI Alliance, the CEPI Alliance and the Bill & Melinda Gates Foundation. It supports research, development and manufacturing of COVID-19 vaccine candidates, negotiates prices and facilitates equitable distribution of vaccines.

Going a step further, India sent a proposal to the WTO in October 2020 for a temporary waiver of the Trade-related Aspects of Intellectual Property Rights provisions.

Knowledge-sharing on a real-time basis was the hallmark of COVID-19 vaccine development efforts. The genome of the contagion was sequenced and published quickly, providing researchers with the genetic instructions for making the spike protein, a key ingredient for developing vaccines. Information-sharing about related coronaviruses, SARS and MERS also helped in saving the critical development time.[32,33]

MULTIPLE NEW TECHNOLOGY PLATFORMS

COVID-19 vaccine development will also be known for the use of novel platform technologies. Messenger RNA (mRNA) was one such platform. It does not require the production of loads of viruses. Scientists only need to know the genetic sequence of a virus to string together the right pieces of the code to synthesize viral antigens in a lab.

When injected, mRNA works as an instruction book for the protein-making machinery in human cells to produce a protein found on the surface of SARS-CoV-2. This spike protein triggers an immune response to the virus.

Earlier, identification of a suitable antigen would take years, but advancements in genomics and structural biology led to the quick mapping of the COVID-19 antigen. This led to the production of the first batch of clinical-grade vaccine material on 7 February 2020, barely four weeks after the publication of the genome sequence. The first dose was administered to a patient on 16 March 2020.

Another novel platform technology used was a viral vector, which was used earlier to develop Ebola vaccines. The RNA sequence of the antigen that triggers an immune response was added to a piece of the genome of a disabled virus to create a vaccine candidate.[32]

FAMILIAR FAMILY: A BIG BOON

The fact that the culprit for the COVID-19 pandemic belonged to the coronavirus family also contributed to the astonishing pace of development of vaccines. SARS-CoV-2 causes an acute disease and stimulates a vanquishing immune response. Therefore, the contagion was an easy target for potential vaccines.[36]

Moreover, the coronavirus family has been studied for decades. Scientists knew that the spike protein of the virus could be targeted by a vaccine. This gave scientists crafting COVID-19 vaccine a head start. The genetic similarity of SARS-CoV-2 with SARS and MERS also gave the scientists a big leg up, and enabled them to quickly rejig ongoing vaccine projects.[34,35]

A SMART HEAD START

Vaccine development involves years of academic research and pre-clinical work, but experience in responding to pandemics such as H1N1, influenza, Ebola, Zika and SARS also comes into use. They led to vaccine development and manufacturing platforms, which are amenable to rapid development of vaccine candidates, swift adaptation as the contagion evolves and fast scale-up of production.

Since these technologies were already in use, prototype vaccines could be developed rapidly. Some safety data on such vaccines existed as well. Next-generation sequencing and reverse genetics have led to a further reduction in the development time of vaccines.

Once SARS-CoV-2 was sequenced, scientists plugged its spike protein's genetic code into a pre-existing technology and came up with the mRNA vaccine candidate within a few days.[38]

The viral vector technology used in some COVID-19 vaccines has been studied for years. It was used to create many vaccines, such as for Ebola, Japanese Encephalitis, SARS, MERS and malaria.[37] Knowledge of this technology aided quick development of COVID-19 vaccines.

Past pandemics have also led to global coordination to respond to infectious diseases. They created global and national infrastructure for vaccine development and production.[37] Researchers relied on innovation in basic genetics, immunology and structural biology to hasten the pace of vaccine development.

SUPERCHARGED FUNDING STREAMS

Vaccine development and production is not just a scientific initiative; it is a money 'guzzler' as well. Therefore, companies do not sink their funds into a new phase of vaccine development before it has been successful in the previous phase. Recognizing this, governments, foundations, philanthropists and other funding agencies went full blast and gave billions of dollars to vaccine developers and manufacturers to draw them into vaccine development. This motivated 'big pharma' in their research and development efforts for development of a vaccine for COVID-19.[37]

Testing is the slowest part of vaccine development. Billions spent on supporting vaccine development made it possible for vaccine companies to conduct efficacy and safety tests on animals and humans at the same time.[37]

But why did this not happen in the case of Ebola? This was because Ebola was devastating poor communities in Africa. Money poured in for the development of a COVID-19 vaccine because this time, it was the wealthy countries that were facing human and economic misery.

THE POWER OF PLENTY

The colossal impact of SARS-CoV-2 and the need to quell it opened up a huge source of funding, which inspired research teams across the globe to join the 'great vaccine hunt'. No one was sure about where a safe and efficacious vaccine would come from. This led to the simultaneous development and testing of hundreds of vaccine candidates with different technologies. It enhanced the probability of development of successful vaccine candidates. The diversity of vaccine candidates made sure that they work in diverse contexts and populations.[39]

ACTING IN PARALLEL, SKIPPING STEPS

The scale and severity of the pandemic required a fast start and steps to be taken in parallel, even without confirming the successful outcome of other steps. Testing in animal models was done simultaneously with clinical trials. Phase-1, Phase-2 and Phase-3 human trials overlapped, speeding up the process.[39] Some trials were collapsed into Phase 1 and 2 or Phase 2 and 3.

Information technology and databases were harnessed in a big way. Epidemiological models were used to identify emerging hot spots and set up clinical sites in these locations to reduce the time for evaluation of the efficacy of vaccines. A control tower strategy was used to monitor the progress of clinical trials.[32] Another novel feature in development of COVID-19 vaccines was that the scientists worked in tandem with the regulators to accelerate the entire process of vaccine development.[40] To hedge the risk of failure, multiple vaccine candidates were developed in parallel.

MANUFACTURING AT RISK

Vaccines not only need money for research and trials, but also to start manufacturing. Since existing vaccine-manufacturing facilities were committed to meet the demand for other routine vaccines, production of COVID-19 vaccines required augmentation of capacity.[39]

Setting up a vaccine-manufacturing plant is expensive. Moreover, a vaccine candidate has only a 20 per cent chance of success, even after reaching the clinical trial stage. Moreover, the pandemic may be over before a vaccine is licensed.[39] Therefore, manufacturers are shy of making such huge investments unless they have a licensed and marketable vaccine. But was this possible in a ravaging pandemic situation?

Deferring expansion of manufacturing facilities then could have led to delays and loss of lives. Hedged for risk by advance orders and financial support, manufacturers pre-built manufacturing facilities and manufacturing was commenced even before the clinical trials were over.[39]

SIZE OF OUTBREAK

The surprisingly fast pace of spread of the contagion was a boon for rapid vaccine development. Vaccine-manufacturing companies need infections to prove the efficacy of their vaccines. Therefore, when a disease itself is not prevalent, efficacy trials become a long-drawn process. In the case of COVID-19, the virus was spreading rapidly. This enabled regulators to quickly verify whether vaccine candidates made a difference.

In Phase-3 trials, tens of thousands of volunteers are needed. However, due to widespread public interest, people enrolled for the trials quickly. Moreover, the virus also affected people in countries with an extensive infrastructure to conduct randomized clinical trials. And because wealthy countries were at the receiving end of the contagion this time, the speed of testing vaccines was accelerated.

REGULATORY NIMBLENESS

Was the rapid journey of vaccines from labs to people's arms possible without the cooperation of national drug regulators? The answer is an emphatic 'no'.

Regulators play a critical role in expediting clinical trials and the final evaluation of the efficacy and safety of a vaccine. COVID-19 witnessed an unprecedented acceleration in the regulatory processes. Regulators mandate more frequent and strong sponsor engagements. National regulators also exchanged information on COVID-19 vaccine trials under the banner 'International Coalition of Medicines Regulatory Authorities'.[35]

Another innovation introduced by many regulators for manufacture of COVID-19 vaccines was a 'rolling review'. This enabled data to be submitted and assessed as it became available. Moreover, EUA provisions were also used liberally. This enabled use of vaccines while the companies were still collecting additional safety- and effectiveness-related information needed for full licensure.[40]

RECORD NUMBER OF VACCINES MADE AVAILABLE IN RECORD TIME

The COVID-19 pandemic spurred an accelerated vaccine development pipeline and saw a rapid growth in the number of vaccines available for use.[41] On 16 March 2020, just two months after the new coronavirus was identified, clinical trials of the first vaccine had commenced. On 24 June 2020, China approved the CanSino vaccine for limited use in the military. The next country to emerge on the vaccine landscape was Russia, which granted emergency use authorization for the Sputnik V vaccine on 11 August 2020. The Pfizer–BioNTech partnership secured temporary regulatory approval in the United Kingdom on 2 December 2020.[37]

As on 19 July 2021, there were 18 vaccines in use and 307 vaccines at different stages of development around the world.[42] The churning out of new vaccines continued throughout 2021. By the beginning of 2022, there were 26 COVID-19 vaccines in use and 308 vaccines at different stages of development.[42] Never in the history of infectious diseases have so many vaccine candidates been at varying stages of development at the same time.

INDIA'S COVID-19 VACCINE DEVELOPMENT JOURNEY: A TRIUMPH OF THE COLLECTIVE

India's role in being the global epicentre for low-cost vaccine manufacturing was critical in producing accessible and affordable vaccines to fight COVID-19. It was also an opportunity to catapult India into a global leadership position in vaccine manufacturing.

The Indian Government responded swiftly by providing an enabling research ecosystem. A National Task Force for Focused Research on COVID-19 vaccines was set up in April 2020. The task force was mandated to guide the process of COVID-19 vaccine development.

A National Biomedical Resource Indigenisation Consortium was set up to converge indigenous resources, products and services for accelerated development of COVID-19 vaccines, diagnostics and therapeutics.

A COVID-19 Vaccine Expert Committee (VEC) was constituted to ensure adoption of a holistic approach in accelerating COVID-19 vaccine development. It also monitored COVID-19 vaccine development projects.

An empowered committee of experts in relevant fields was constituted to facilitate and guide applicants on regulatory requirements. It was also decided to fast track the regulatory approval process. To do this, timelines for each step were prescribed.

Addressing the nation on the occasion of Independence Day 2020, the India's Prime Minister Narendra Modi said 'I would like to tell my countrymen that our scientists are dutifully engaged in the laboratories. They are putting in great efforts. At present, testing for three vaccines is at different stages in the country'.

To further speed up vaccine manufacturing in India, and in view of research-related collaboration between Indian companies and foreign research organizations, it was decided to consider preclinical studies already conducted outside India for regulatory submission. Applicants were also provided facilities to submit parallel applications to conduct the appropriate phases of trials.

Although the extant statutory provisions lacked explicit provisions regarding public health emergencies or provisions for granting EUA, the Indian regulator responded to the unmet need and allowed 'restricted emergency use'.

Prime Minister, Narendra Modi led the vaccine research and development programme from the front. He facilitated a conducive environment for vaccine manufacturers to encourage accelerated research and development and manufacture of vaccines in the spirit of Atmanirbhar Bharat. In the midst of the pandemic, he visited the vaccine-manufacturing facilities. He directly engaged with manufacturers and motivated them to produce the much needed vaccines quickly.

The Indian government also supported indigenous vaccine manufacturers financially. During interactions, Rajesh Bhushan, the Union Health Secretary, told me: 'The Government of India has provided 100% advance payment to domestic vaccine manufacturers for procurement orders placed with them. These funds can be used by the manufacturers for capacity augmentation'. On 23 April 2021 the Ministry of Health informed the Parliament that one of the domestic vaccine manufacturers was also given financial assistance for 'at-risk manufacturing' of COVID-19 vaccine.

There were challenges posed by shortage of raw materials and consumables due to the surge in the global demand and the consequent imposition of statutory control on exports by their producing countries. The critical raw materials included filters, single-use bioreactor bags, culture media, excipients, tubing, cartridges, resins for filtration and adjuvants.

'We interacted with the vaccine manufacturers, identified raw materials with a high degree of dependence and contacted source countries such as the USA, the United Kingdom, Germany, France, Singapore and Japan. We looked for and encouraged domestic manufacturers as well', said Dr Yuvraj, Joint Secretary Pharmaceuticals. As a long-term measure, APIs and other critical raw materials for vaccine manufacturing were included in the government's PLI scheme to make India self-sufficient. Under the scheme, an incentive of 10 per cent was provided for incremental sales of these products.

When finally, the vaccines were ready to be rolled out, everyone was ecstatic. Prime Minister Modi said to the Chief Ministers of all the states in a meeting on 11 January 2021, 'It is a matter of pride for all of us that the two vaccines that have been given emergency use authorization are both made in India'.

Thirty other Indian companies had also embarked on the journey of developing COVID-19 vaccines. Many of them were supported by the Government of India.

From the beginning, India made it clear that its vaccines would be made available to the entire world. Addressing the 75th United Nations General Assembly Session 2020, Prime Minister Modi said: 'India's vaccine production and delivery capacity will be used to help all humanity in fighting this crisis'. At the Invest India Conference in Canada the following month, the Prime Minister reiterated his commitment: 'We want to help the entire world when it comes to vaccine production for Covid-19'.

MISSION COVID SURAKSHA: INDIA'S COVID-19 VACCINE DEVELOPMENT MISSION

The Government of India launched its mission COVID Suraksha as a part of the third economic stimulus package under Atmanirbhar Bharat to bring the economy, battered by the COVID-19 pandemic, back on track. The mission aims to produce safe, efficacious and affordable COVID-19 vaccines with the preferred characteristics applicable to India. The objective of the mission is to accelerate the development of five to six vaccine candidates so that two to four of them are licensed and marketed.

The mission is being implemented by BIRAC, a public sector undertaking (PSU) of the DBT.

It is supporting the establishment of clinical trial sites, immune assay laboratories and facilities for animal challenge studies. It is also funding manufacturing and testing facilities, training, data management systems, regulatory submissions, quality management and accreditation.

According to the Department of Biotechnology of the Government of India, under the Mission, the Department has endeavoured to build a new vaccine development ecosystem. In its first year, the Mission provided financial support amounting to ₹4.07 billion to vaccine candidates of Zydus Cadila for its ZyCoVD vaccine, to Biological E for its Corbevax vaccine, to Bharat Biotech for its BBV-154 vaccine, to Gennova Biopharmaceuticals for its HGCO-19 vaccine and to Genique Lifesciences for its VLP vaccine. In addition, the mission provided financial assistance of ₹528.16 million to enhance the capacities of five animal challenge studies and support the immune-assay laboratories of three vaccine manufacturers.

The Department confirmed that it has spent ₹318.22 million on supporting 19 pan-India good clinical research practice-compliant-related clinical trial sites. Moreover, it provided ₹2.2 billion to Bharat Biotech to augment its manufacture of Covaxin and funds to three PSUs to scale up their production of Covaxin. The PSUs supported by the mission are Haffkine Biopharmaceutical Corporation Ltd, Indian Immunologicals Limited and Bharat Immunologicals Biologicals Limited.

Under the DBT's Resource of Indian Vaccine Epidemiology Network, 11 GCLP-compliant clinical trial sites have been established to facilitate quick clinical trials. Each site has access to around 50,000–100,000 healthy volunteers.

DBT-BIRAC has also facilitated the transfer of production technology for Covaxin to the Gujarat COVID Vaccine Consortium. The consortium comprises Hester Biosciences, OmniBRx Biotechnologies Pvt. Ltd and Gujarat Biotechnology Research Centre. The efforts were aimed at increasing production of Covaxin from 10 million doses per month to 100 million doses per month.

According to Dr Jyoti Logani, Scientist, DBT, the department's laboratories at the National Institute of Animal Biotechnology (NIAB) in Hyderabad and the National Centre for Cell Science (NCCS) in Pune were also upgraded to become Central Drug Laboratories (CDLs). 'The department has also set up vaccine-testing facilities at DBT-NCCS and DBT-NIAB with the support of the PM-CARES Fund', she said.

₹900 crore was allocated to the Mission for 12 months. The government also allocated ₹100 crore from the PM-CARES Fund to support vaccine-development initiatives.[43]

India's Ministry of External Affairs and DBT joined hands to build clinical trial capacity in neighbouring Lower Middle Income Countries (LMICs) Partnering countries were granted access to the Indian vaccine-development ecosystem, for instance, immunogenicity assay testing of potential vaccine candidates.

Training programmes were also organized to strengthen the clinical trial research capacity in neighbouring countries. These programmes were attended by participants from Afghanistan, Bahrain, Bhutan, Bangladesh, Gambia, Kenya, Myanmar, Maldives, Mauritius, Oman, Nepal, Somalia, Sri Lanka and Vietnam.

PRIVATE SECTOR EFFORTS FOR VACCINE DEVELOPMENT

Many Indian vaccine manufacturers collaborated with global and Indian organizations on tech-transfer, co-development and manufacturing of COVID-19 vaccines. Their efforts paid off handsomely.

On 4 January 2021, India's regulator approved restricted use of two COVID-19 vaccines, Covaxin and Covishield, in emergency situations. This marked India's entry into the five COVID-19 vaccine-producing countries. The USA, the United Kingdom, Russia and China were the other countries in this club.

Thereafter, many more private Indian vaccine manufacturers, including Cedilla Healthcare, Biological E. and Panacea Biotech, rolled out COVID-19 vaccines in 2021.

India's Health Secretary, Rajesh Bhushan, while talking to me, attributed India's success in developing COVID-19 vaccines to the leadership of Prime Minister Modi and incessant efforts made under the Atmanirbhar Bharat scheme. He also thanked the Indian vaccine manufacturers for rising to the occasion and producing impressive results.

COVISHIELD: A PRODUCT OF INTERNATIONAL COLLABORATION

The British-Swedish company AstraZeneca and Oxford University developed a non-replicating viral vector COVID-19 vaccine.[40] The SII signed an agreement with the developers in June 2020 to collaborate in development, manufacturing and distribution of the potential vaccine.[40] The Indian government extended a helping hand by reforming regulatory pathways to cut short the approval timeline.[44] SII also entered into an agreement to produce the Novavax COVID-19 vaccine.

COVAXIN: INDIA'S FIRST FULLY INDIGENOUS COVID-19 VACCINE

In March 2020, ICMR scientists isolated the SARS-CoV-2 virus. India became the fifth country in the world to achieve this feat. The ICMR collaborated with Bharat Biotech Ltd on development of a vaccine.[44] They developed a whole-virion inactivated vaccine.[40] The technology is also used to manufacture vaccines for influenza, rabies and hepatitis A.[40] In January 2021, the vaccine got approval for 'restricted use in emergencies under the clinical trial mode' pending Phase-3 clinical trial data. Although this invited criticism initially, the vaccine has made a vital contribution to India's fight against COVID-19.

All Indian vaccines licensed till the writing of this book are suitable for use in India. They can be stored in ordinary refrigerators at 2–8° degrees Celsius. They can be transported at +20–+8 degrees Celsius.[40] On the other hand, foreign-made COVID-19 vaccines by major manufacturers must be stored at –70° Celsius. Indian vaccines are also significantly cheaper than their foreign counterparts. Therefore, they are destined to be the saviours of the people of LMICs.

INDIA'S VACCINE STORE

Apart from Covaxin and Covishield, India has many more vaccines in its COVID-19 vaccine store. Moreover, the Indian government has fast-tracked approval of vaccines that are already licensed for emergency use by international bodies and other regulators.

The CDSCO has granted emergency use authorization for the imported Sputnik V, as well as for the Moderna and Johnson & Johnson vaccines. This has expanded India's COVID-19 vaccine basket to five vaccines. On 20 August 2021, India created history by approving the world's first DNA COVID-19 vaccine for emergency use. Named ZyCoV-D, the vaccine is manufactured by Cadila Healthcare and was developed in partnership with the DBT under COVID Suraksha mission. The SII's Covovax and Biological E.'s Corbevax were the next to secure approval on 28 December 2021. Corbevax is a subunit vaccine.

Thus, by the end of 2021, India had a bouquet of 7 COVID-19 vaccines approved for emergency use. With many other Indian vaccines in clinical trials, India's COVID-19 vaccine basket is set to bulge in the year 2022.

The vaccines under development include Gennova Biopharmaceuticals' mRNA vaccine, HGCO19; Bharat Biotech's intranasal vaccine, BBV154; Intas' Novel Active Virosome of the Seagull recombinant adeno-associated virus vaccine; Genique's VLP vaccine, and SII's repurposed BCG vaccine, which are in various stages of clinical trials. In addition, many other vaccine candidates are in their early or advanced pre-clinical trial phases. The single-dose intranasal COVID-19 vaccine being developed by Bharat Biotech in collaboration with Washington University School of Medicine in St. Louis is believed to be a game changer because of its numerous advantages.

The COVID-19 pandemic has demonstrated that vaccines can be developed against new diseases at a stunning speed. It has shown the world the way to deal with future pandemics and fight existing vaccine-preventable diseases. In the next chapter, I will elaborate on the world's largest vaccination drive that India has embarked on to defeat SARS-CoV-2.

REFERENCES

1. Listings of WHO's response to COVID-19 [Internet]. WHO.int. 2021 [cited 31 July 2021]. Available from: https://www.who.int/news/item/29-06-2020-covidtimeline
2. Wu YC, Chen CS, Chan YJ. The outbreak of COVID-19: An overview. *Journal of the Chinese Medical Association*. 2020 March;83(3):217.
3. WHO statement regarding cluster of pneumonia cases in Wuhan, China [Internet]. WHO.int. 2021 [cited 31 July 2021]. Available from: https://www.who.int/china/news/detail/09-01-2020-who-statement-regarding-cluster-of-pneumonia-cases-in-wuhan-china
4. Novel coronavirus (2019-nCoV) situation report. 21 January 2020. WHO.int. 2021 [cited 31 July 2021]. Available from: https://www.who.int/docs/default-source/coronaviruse/situation-reports/20200121-sitrep-1-2019-ncov.pdf
5. WHO coronavirus (COVID-19) dashboard [Internet]. Covid19.who.int. 2021 [cited 31 July 2021]. Available from: https://covid19.who.int/
6. MoHFW. Home [Internet]. Mohfw.gov.in. 2021 [cited 31 July 2021]. Available from: https://www.mohfw.gov.in/
7. World Health Organization. WHO-convened global study of origins of SARS-CoV-2: China Part.
8 Lu D. The hunt to find the coronavirus pandemic's patient zero. *New Scientist* (1971). 2020 April 4;245(3276):9.

9. Huang C, Wang Y, Li X, Ren L, Zhao J, Hu Y, Zhang L, et al. Clinical features of patients infected with 2019 novel coronavirus in Wuhan, China. *The Lancet*. 2020 February 15;395(10223):497–506.
10. Leung GM, Leung K. Crowdsourcing data to mitigate epidemics. *The Lancet Digital Health*. 2020 April 1;2(4):e156-7.
11. Li X, Zai J, Wang X, Li Y. Potential of large 'first generation' human-to-human transmission of 2019-nCoV. *Journal of Medical Virology*. 2020 April;92(4):448–454.
12. Wuhan lab staff went to hospital before COVID-19 outbreak was disclosed: Report. *The Wire*, Science [Internet]. *The Wire Science*. 2021 [cited 31 July 2021]. Available from: https://science.thewire.in/health/wuhan-lab-staff-hospital-covid-19-origins/
13. Origin of Covid-19: Why Wuhan lab in China continues to be prime suspect [Internet]. *India Today*. 2021 [cited 31 July 2021]. Available from: *https://www.indiatoday.in/coronavirus-outbreak/story/covid-19-origin-wuhan-lab-china-britain-us-investigation-1809059-2021-05-31*
14. Seventy-third world health assembly agenda item-3. 18 May 2020. COVID-19 response. Apps.who.int. 2021 [cited 31 July 2021]. Available from: https://apps.who.int/gb/ebwha/pdf_files/WHA73/A73_CONF1Rev1-en.pdf
15. We may never find 'patient zero' of Covid-19: WHO [Internet]. @businessline. 2021 [cited 31 July 2021]. Available from: https://www.thehindubusinessline.com/news/science/we-may-never-find-patient-zero-of-covid-19-who/article33607229.ece
16. Drew H, McKay B. WHO report into Covid-19 origins leaves key questions unanswered [Internet]. WSJ. 2021 [cited 31 July 2021]. Available from: https://www.wsj.com/articles/who-report-into-covid-19-origins-leaves-key-questions-unanswered-11617027920
17. Wilkie C, R Mendez. Biden orders closer review of Covid origins as U.S. intel weighs Wuhan lab leak theory. [Internet]. 2021 [cited 31 July 2021]. Available from: **https://www.cnbc.com/2021/05/26/biden-orders-us-intelligence-to-intensify-investigation-into-covid-19-origins.html**
18. Laskar R H. India backs WHO chief's call for further investigations into Covid-19 origin [Internet]. *Hindustan Times*. 2021 [cited 31 July 2021]. Available from: **https://www.hindustantimes.com/india-news/india-responds-to-who-study-on-covid-19-origin-calls-for-comprehensive-mechanism-101617295739356.html**
19. Kramer J, 2021. Here's what the WHO report found on the origins of COVID-19. National Geographic. https://www.nationalgeographic.com/science/article/heres-what-the-who-report-found-on-the-origins-Covid-19
20. Regalado A. No one can find the animal that gave people Covid-19 [Internet]. *MIT Technology Review*. 2021 [cited 31 July 2021]. Available

from: https://www.technologyreview.com/2021/03/26/1021263/bat-covid-coronavirus-cause-origin-wuhan/

21. What do we know about investigation into Covid origin: All you need to know [Internet]. *Times of India*. 2021 [cited 31 July 2021] Available from: https://timesofindia.indiatimes.com/world/us/what-do-we-know-about-investigation-into-covid-origin-all-you-need-to-know/articleshow/83429101.cms
22. Mishra A. Significant evidence that Covid originated from Wuhan lab [Internet] *Sunday Guardian* Live. 2021 [cited 31 July 2021] Available from: https://www.sundayguardianlive.com/news/significant-evidence-covid-originated-wuhan-lab
23. Ghosh P. Is Wuhan's 'Patient Su' Covid's patient zero? Report reveals new timeline of infection. [Internet]. *Hindustan Times*. [cited 31 July 2021] Available from: https://www.hindustantimes.com/world-news/is-wuhan-s-patient-su-covid-s-patient-zero-report-reveals-new-timeline-of-infection-101622360922716.html
24. Researchers from Wuhan lab sought hospital care before Covid-19 outbreak disclosed: Report. [Internet]. *ANI News*. [Cited 31 July 2021]. Available from: https://www.aninews.in/news/world/asia/researchers-from-wuhan-lab-sought-hospital-care-before-covid-19-outbreak-disclosed-report20210524095126/
25. British Intelligence believes Covid-19 lab leak theory 'feasible': Report. [Internet] *Business Standard* [Cited 31 July 2021. Available from: https://www.business-standard.com/article/international/british-intelligence-believes-covid-19-lab-leak-theory-feasible-report-121053000903_1.html
26. Wade N. The origin of COVID: Did people or nature open Pandora's box at Wuhan. *Bulletin of the Atomic Scientists*. 2021. Available from: https://thebulletin.org/2021/05/the-origin-of-covid-did-people-or-nature-open-pandoras-box-at-wuhan/
27. Ghosh, A. Wuhan lab's deleted data, unreported pneumonia cases: Challenges to 'natural' origins of Covid. 4 June 2021. Available from: https://theprint.in/science/wuhan-labs-deleted-data-unreported-pneumonia-cases-challenges-to-natural-origins-of-covid/671984/
28. Niewijk G. Controversy aside, why the source of COVID-19 matters. *Geneng News*. 21 September 2020. Available from: https://www.genengnews.com/insights/controversy-aside-why-the-source-of-covid-19-matters/
29. A coordinated global research roadmap: 2019 novel coronavirus. WHO [Internet] 2021. [cited 31 July 2021] Available from: https://www.who.int/blueprint/priority-diseases/key-action/Coronavirus_Roadmap_V9.pdf
30. Pregelj L, Hine DC, Oyola-Lozada MG, Munro TP. Working hard or hardly working? Regulatory bottlenecks in developing a COVID-19 vaccine. *Trends in Biotechnology*. 2020 September 1;38(9):943–947.
31. How did the COVID-19 vaccine get developed so quickly? [Internet] 2021 [cited 31 July 2021. Available from: https://portal.ct.gov/-/media/

Coronavirus/Community_Resources/Vaccinations/Print-Materials/Fact-Sheets/Development_English.pdf

32. Fast-forward: Will the speed of COVID-19 vaccine development reset industry norms? McKinsey & Company. [Internet] 2021 [cited 31 July 2021. Available from: **https://www.mckinsey.com/industries/life-sciences/our-insights/fast-forward-will-the-speed-of-covid-19-vaccine-development-reset-industry-norms**
33. Byrd A. How the COVID-19 vaccines were made so quickly—from the lab to clinical trials to FDA Authorization. Explore Health. [Internet] 2021. [cited 31 July 2021]. Available from: https://www.health.com/condition/infectious-diseases/coronavirus/how-covid-19-vaccine-was-made-quickly
34. McCallum K. How was the COVID-19 vaccine developed so fast? *Houston Methodist*. [Internet] 2021 [cited 31 July 2021] Available from: https://www.houstonmethodist.org/blog/articles/2020/dec/how-was-the-covid-19-vaccine-developed-so-fast/
35. Cassata C. Here's how it was possible to develop COVID-19 vaccines so quickly. *Healthline*. [Internet] 2021 [cited 31 July 2021] Available from: https://www.healthline.com/health-news/heres-how-it-was-possible-to-develop-covid-19-vaccines-so-quickly
36. Joseph A. A huge experiment: How the world made so much progress on a Covid-19 vaccine so fast. Statnews [Internet] 2021 [cited 31 July 2021]. Available from: https://www.statnews.com/2020/07/30/a-huge-experiment-how-the-world-made-so-much-progress-on-a-covid-19-vaccine-so-fast/
37. Ball P. The lightning-fast quest for COVID vaccines—and what it means for other diseases. *Nature*. [Internet] 2021 [cited 31 July 2021] Available from: https://www.nature.com/articles/d41586-020-03626-1
38. Were the COVID-19 vaccines rushed? Here's how the vaccines were developed so fast. *Nebraska Medicine*. [Internet] 2021 [cited 31 July 2021.Available from: https://www.nebraskamed.com/COVID/were-the-covid-19-vaccines-rushed
39. How did scientists manage to develop safe COVID-19 vaccines in just ten months? GAVI. *The Vaccine Alliance*. [Internet] 2021 [cited 31 July 2021] Available from: https://www.gavi.org/vaccineswork/how-did-scientists-manage-develop-safe-covid-19-vaccines-just-ten-months
40. FAQs for healthcare workers and front-line workers. Ministry of Health and Family Welfare Government of India. [Internet] 2021 [cited 31 July 2021] Available from https://www.mohfw.gov.in/
41. Krammer F. SARS-CoV-2 vaccines in development. *Nature*. 2020 October;586(7830):516–527.
42. COVID-19 vaccine tracker. London School of Hygiene and Tropical Medicine. [Internet] 2021 [cited 31 July 2021] Available from: https://vac-lshtm.shinyapps.io/ncov_vaccine_landscape/
43. Dutt A. Indian Covid-19 vaccine development to be backed by PM-CARES Fund. *Hindustan Times* [Internet] 2021 [cited 31 July 2021]. Available from:

https://www.hindustantimes.com/india-news/indian-vaccine-development-to-be-backed-by-pm-cares/story-RLUxmlAlPnheClpTLbaSEK.html
44. Kapoor A. India's vaccine development journey: A triumph of the collective. *The Economic Times* [Internet] 2021 [cited 31 July 2021] Available from: https://economictimes.indiatimes.com/industry/healthcare/biotech/healthcare/indias-vaccine-development-journey-a-triumph-of-the-collective/articleshow/83788567.cms?from=mdr

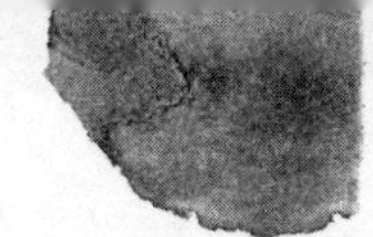

Chapter 6

World's Biggest Vaccination Drive

Soon after joining the elite club of COVID-19 vaccine producers, India embarked on the world's largest and fastest vaccination drive. However, the big question is: how did India manage to do it?

VAST EXPERIENCE OF MASS VACCINATION

India has had vast experience of running mass vaccination campaigns in the past. Apart from the eradication of smallpox and polio through mass vaccination drives under its UIP, India has administered 390 million vaccines annually to pregnant women and children.[1,2]

India also had a trained workforce of 2.5 million health workers and 50,000 cold chain technicians (CCTs) to handle its UIP. An extensive countrywide cold chain network was available for routine immunization as well.

However, could India's success in routine immunization guarantee the same victory in its massive COVID-19 vaccination drive?

A MISSION FRAUGHT WITH FORMIDABLE CHALLENGES

India's COVID-19 vaccination campaign was unique in terms of its scale of operations, delivery timelines, infrastructural requirements and the large number of people needing immunization.

While talking to me, Chesta Yadav, the District Magistrate of Delhi's North-West district, admitted that 'the scale of COVID vaccination was huge in contrast to the target population for routine immunization'. While the UIP was confined mostly to government health facilities, the scale of COVID-19 vaccinations required vaccination centres to operate in other public and private spaces as well, she told me.

In addition, the campaign necessitated large-scale adult immunization, hitherto not usual in India. Another daunting challenge was the rapid pace of vaccination to cover 1.4 billion people within the span of months needed to see the back of the pandemic.[1] Apart from availability of vaccines, rapid expansion of cold chain and other logistics, mobilization of human resources and their training were critical.

Transporting vaccines at the right temperature was a gigantic task. 'This was especially daunting in the remote and hilly areas of the country,' said Dr Devansh Yadav, Deputy Commissioner, Changlang district of Arunachal Pradesh during interactions. The hilly district, with a dense forest cover, a tiger reserve, and numerous rivers and streams, is spread over 4,500 square kilometres.

Prioritization of target groups, dealing with vaccine hesitancy and eagerness, preventing misinformation, building community ownership and generating a demand for vaccines are other challenges that needed to be tackled. Dr A. Muthamma, Health Secretary of Dadra and Nagar Haveli and Daman and Diu, rated 'the apprehensions of citizens regarding the safety and efficacy of the vaccine' as the most formidable challenge.

'Uploading data about healthcare workers on the CoWIN portal in the initial phase was a huge challenge in a large part of Arunachal Pradesh due to the lack of a stable internet connection', Dr P. Parthiban, Health Secretary of the state told me. This was reiterated by Akhil Arora, Principle Secretary, Health, Government of Rajasthan. 'People in rural areas have limited accessibility and understanding of the portal,' he confided.

So how did India overcome these challenges?

EFFECTIVE COORDINATION AND FAST-TRACKING DECISIONS

According to India's Health Secretary, Rajesh Bhushan, 'excellent cooperation and coordination with all stakeholders, including various ministries of the union government, state governments, development partners, non-governmental organizations and civil society organizations, was a critical factor'. To make the drive a success, the Government of India adopted a whole-government and whole-society approach for the vaccination drive, he told me.

A robust governance mechanism was designed for effective coordination and swift decision-making. At the national level, the National Expert Group on Vaccine Administration for COVID-19 (NEGVAC) provided regulatory guidance on vaccine trials, planning of vaccine administration, inter-sectoral coordination, financing, procurement and distribution, prioritization of population groups, supply chain infrastructure, vaccine safety surveillance, community engagement and awareness generation.[3] In the states, a state-level steering committee headed by the Chief Secretary was assigned the policy guidance, coordination and oversight functions. A state-level task force was made responsible for planning and mapping vaccination sessions, strengthening cold chain infrastructure, identifying manpower, training and managing bio-medical waste, developing a media plan to allay fears and misinformation, attracting people to vaccination centres and monitoring their progress.

A District Task Force functions under the District Magistrate in every district. Similar task forces were also set up at the block and municipal levels. 'Island-level Monitoring Committees were constituted under the chairmanship of the Deputy Collector',

Amit Satija, Health Secretary of Lakshadweep, told me during an interaction. Lakshadweep is a federally administered territory of India comprising 36 small islands, many of which are uninhabited.

LEVERAGING ELECTORAL EXPERIENCE OF THE WORLD'S LARGEST DEMOCRACY

If there is one task of the same scale and complexity that India undertakes with perfection, ironically, it is the conduct of elections. More than one million polling stations are set up and five million workers are deployed to reach more than 900 million voters for general elections to Lok Sabha. The process is completed in a span of weeks.

Managers of the COVID-19 vaccination programme drew heavily on the expertise, experience and infrastructure for conducting elections. Voter rolls were used to identify eligible people and decide on the location of vaccination centres.

Designing of vaccination centres, deployment of staff and flow of people were all based on the pattern of an election booth. Like polling day responsibilities, the role of each member of a vaccination team was precisely defined. Chesta Yadav, who had the formidable target of vaccinating 1.6 million people with two doses by the end of 2021, told me, 'We went back to our most trusted and reliable system—the conduct of elections'. She also told me that setting up of vaccination centres at polling locations, training of manpower, ensuring the safety of vaccines, and so forth, were all accomplished with the same rigor and precision as conducting the elections.

Co-WIN: THE DIGITAL VACCINE ADMINISTRATOR

Administering 390 million vaccine doses annually under India's UIP is in itself an epic mission. Therefore, in 2015, a web-based system called the Electronic Vaccine Intelligence Network (eVIN) was developed. Through a smartphone application, eVIN provided real-time information on availability of vaccine stocks and the storage temperature across all cold chain points (CCPs) in the country.[4] Necessary training was also imparted to people involved in the process.[5]

In the second half of 2020, when the Ministry of Health and Family Welfare started planning the vaccination drive, it was decided to adopt an end-to-end digital approach to manage the vaccine inventory, and cold chain and vaccine administration. 'Since each vaccine was precious, it was necessary that each dose was tracked and wastage was minimized', the Prime Minister Modi later told a global conclave on 5 July 2021. Moreover, it was necessary to provide an easily accessible record to people of when and where and by whom they had been vaccinated.

This led to efforts being made for reincarnation of eVIN, which was named Co-WIN, and became the technological backbone of the National COVID-19 Vaccination Programme. The reincarnation resulted in many new modules such as beneficiary registration and management, vaccine distribution, logistic management, session site planning, team allotment, vaccine scheduling, generation of vaccination certificates and adverse events following immunization (AEFI) monitoring.[6]

Co-WIN is a cloud-based, open source, scalable, online platform developed by the central government. It is used by all stakeholders starting from the national team in New Delhi to the state teams, district administration and down to the individual vaccinators.[7,8]

Rajesh Bhushan told me more about Co-WIN. He said, 'This indigenous web portal was developed in record time and enabled real-time monitoring of the status of a vaccination drive, and availability and utilization of vaccines'. Co-WIN's beneficiary management module was used for registration of beneficiaries, provision of information on the schedule of sessions, as well as the availability and price of vaccines; scheduling of vaccination appointments and generation of vaccination certificates.[3,9]

According to the affidavit filed by Dr Manohar Agnani, Additional Secretary, Ministry of Health and Family Welfare, Government of India, in the Supreme Court of India in June 2021, a common portal to capture and maintain the digital footprint of vaccination had numerous advantages. It provided verifiable data on the number of citizens vaccinated, ensured that people received the second dose of the same vaccine, maintained the required time gap between the first and the second dose, and prevented administration of more than the prescribed number of doses as well as pilferages.[10]

He also said that the system provided vaccination certificates to vaccinated persons, which can be accessed anytime from anywhere. Co-WIN enabled administrators and Programme Managers to monitor the progress of vaccination overall and for specific geographical segments, check the availability and utilization of vaccines and plan future vaccination programmes, assess wastage of vaccines and take measures to minimize it and formulate policies.[10]

In the spirit of *vasudhaiva kusudhaiva* (the whole world is my family), India even offered this digital platform to all countries, along with the necessary technical assistance, to help them conduct their vaccination drives.

Speaking at the Co-WIN Global Conclave on 5 July 2021, Prime Minister Modi said, 'Indian civilization considers the whole world as one family. That's why, our technology platform Co-WIN is being prepared to be made open source and will be available to any and all countries'.

According to Mr Bhushan, more than 100 countries had shown an interest for uptake and operationalization of Co-WIN for their vaccination drives. India's Ministry of Health and Family Welfare also joined the WHO's COVID-19 Technology Access Pool

(C-TAP) initiative by sharing India's Co-WIN Platform on WHO C-TAP. However, Co-WIN is yet to be adopted by any country. However, use of Co-WIN pan-India is the only way to register oneself for vaccination and conduct vaccine drives and has its own challenges. The formidable ones are the lack of availability of hardware, trained manpower and internet connectivity.

STRENGTHENING THE COLD CHAIN

Temperature-controlled equipment and procedures maintain the potency and safety of vaccines. For UIP, India has set up an extensive countrywide cold chain network from where vaccines are taken to eight million vaccination sites.[2] However, the COVID-19 vaccination drive needs a substantial augmentation of the cold chain capacity.[11]

As per Dr Manohar Agnani, there are 29,116 CCPs across the country where the vaccines are stored at recommended temperatures. These include four national-level stores, 37 state vaccine stores, 114 regional vaccine stores, 723 district vaccine stores and 28,268 sub-district vaccine stores. CCPs have cold chain equipment (CCE) such as walk-in-coolers (WICs), walk-in-freezers (WIFs), ice lined refrigerators (ILRs), deep freezers (DFs) and cold boxes for storage of vaccines and freezing of icepacks.[10]

The Indian government informed Parliament on 23 July 2021 that a detailed analysis of cold chain infrastructure across the country was carried out prior to the introduction of the COVID-19 vaccine for enhancement and augmentation. The requirement of passive CCE such as cold boxes, vaccine carriers, temperature loggers and vaccine vial monitors was also assessed.[3]

As per Dr Agnani, the Government of India centrally procured CCE and supplied it to the states. The number of WICs was increased from 243 in March 2020 to 280 by June 2021, WIFs from 73 to 103, ILRs from 41,985 to 50,529, DFs from 39,036 to 54,101 and cold boxes from 60,405 to 69,650. Moreover, funds were allocated to the states under the National Health Mission (NHM) for maintenance of CCEs and hiring of CCTs for their repair and maintenance.[10]

State-wide, rigorous monitoring of CCPs was undertaken to estimate the cold chain and other logistic requirements for the drive. 'Deficiencies were immediately corrected and reviewed', shared Akhil Arora, Principle Secretary of Health, Rajasthan. Training programmes for CCTs and managers on cold chain and vaccine management were also organized.

District magistrates were asked to review existing cold chain infrastructure in their districts. This was augmented based on local conditions and requirements. 'Remote areas with no electricity were provided standalone solar ILRs for vaccine storage', said Dr Devansh.

State governments pitched in as well, said Mayur Dixit, District Magistrate of Uttarkashi in Uttarakhand. Available equipment was repaired, said Bhaskar Katamneni, Mission Director, NHM, Andhra Pradesh. Customized refrigerators, which can maintain their temperature from 2° to 8° Celsius for several days in the event of a power failure, were designed.[1,2]

MEETING THE TRANSPORTATION CHALLENGE: TRAVERSING AIR, WATER AND LAND

Transportation of vaccines in temperature-controlled facilities through the vast expanse of India was a challenge. Vaccines travel thousands of miles by aeroplanes, trucks, trains and foot. People waded through geographically inaccessible areas, difficult hilly terrain, snow-clad mountains and thick forests. Special emphasis was laid on the safety and security of each dose, with a 24 × 7 deployment of security personnel at vaccine storage points during their transportation and at vaccination sites.

Rajesh Bhushan elaborated on the arrangements made: 'To reduce transportation hours, we followed a policy of door delivery of vaccines by suppliers through refrigerated vans that maintained the approved temperature benchmark for COVID-19 vaccines to designated consignee points.' The cost was included in the cost of the vaccine. 'The number of consignee points across India was increased from 41 to 60. This reduced transportation hours substantially.' He added, 'We already had temperature-controlled transportation in place for UIP'.

However, according to the state governments, the transportation of vaccines at the desired temperature was a huge challenge. Bhaskar said: 'There was a shortage of refrigerated vehicles to meet the demand. In addition to existing fleets, private refrigerated vehicles were hired to transport vaccines from the state vaccine stores to regional vaccine stores and districts, and to PHCs and all CCPs'.

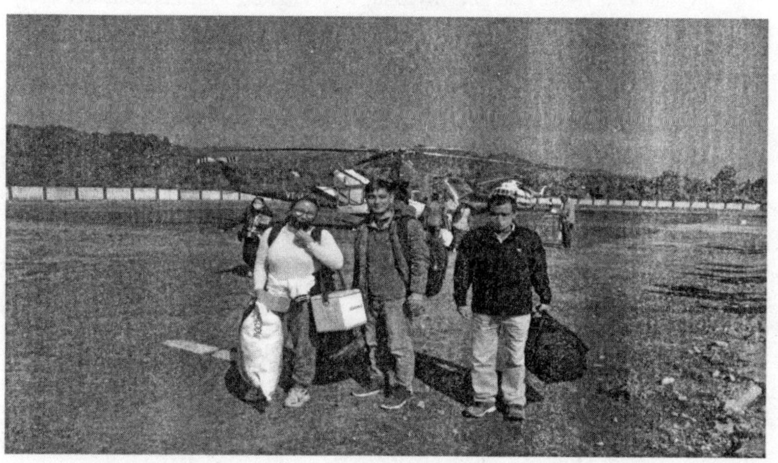

Vaccination Teams in Arunachal Pradesh Had to Take Aerial Route

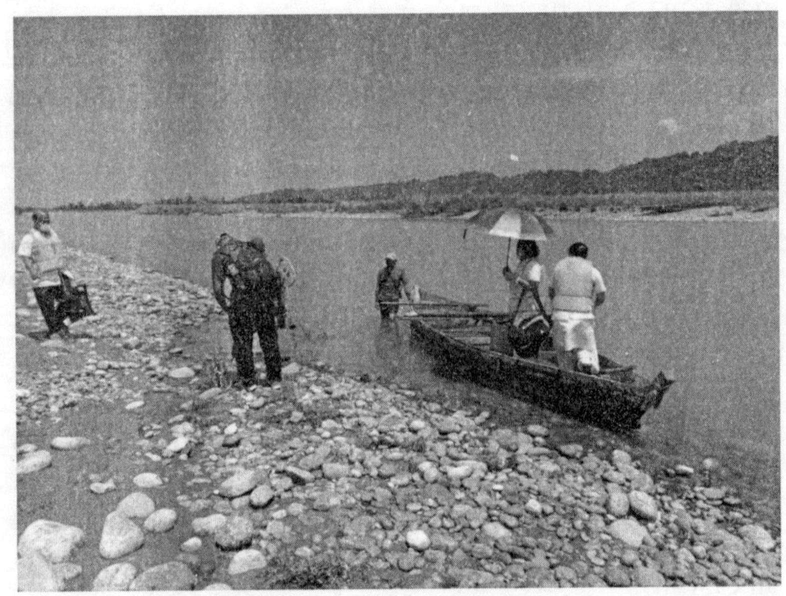

Vaccination Teams Had to Cross Many Rivers to Reach Their Destination

Dr P. Parthiban, Health Secretary of Arunachal Pradesh, located in the northeast corner of India on the Indo-China border, seconded him, 'Transportation of vaccines to hard-to-reach areas was a big challenge. We had to deploy helicopters to cut down the transportation time'.

Dr Devansh, who had an uphill task in one of the remotest districts in India, told me: 'We transported vaccines and vaccination teams by boats, JCBs, excavators and on foot. We had to make temporary hanging bridges of cane and bamboo for the teams to cross rivers'. ICMR came up with a drone project to transport vaccines to inaccessible health facilities in Manipur.

A LOGISTICAL NIGHTMARE

Another Herculean task was arranging the logistics of dispensing vaccines. These included ancillary items such as auto-disabled syringes, needles, glass vials, alcohol swabs, hub-cutters, biomedical waste bags and so forth.[8]

Along with vaccines, the Central Ministry of Health and Family Welfare initiated procurement of syringes and other necessary items. Rajesh Bhushan told me about the arrangements made. He said: 'We initiated procurement of syringes for COVID-19 in 2020. Availability of syringes and requirement projections were continuously reviewed and aligned with revised vaccination policies'.

Fresh tenders were floated, including a global tender in July 2021 for the procurement of the required number of syringes for the large number of people to be vaccinated. 'Regular meetings were conducted under the chairperson and senior officials for frontloading as well as timely supply of syringes', Rajesh Bhushan explained. Dedicated dry storage space for syringes and other requirements was also arranged in vaccine stores at various levels.[3]

Despite all this, however, some states reported shortage of syringes at the peak of their vaccination drives. 'Shortage of auto-disposable syringes was experienced a few times during the vaccination drive and these had to be procured by the state', admitted Bhaskar. Initially, Auto Disposable (AD) syringes of 0.5 ml were being used for COVID-19 vaccination in government facilities. However, to meet the shortage of syringes, the government decided to use syringes of other sizes: 1 ml, 2 ml and 3 ml.

An equally formidable task was disposal of the huge quantities of biomedical waste generated.

IDENTIFICATION OF VACCINATION CENTRES

The responsibility of identifying vaccination centres was assigned to the District Magistrates. Multi-disciplinary teams were formed to identify suitable vaccination sites. 'We used PHCs, community health centres, community halls, schools and government offices to establish CVCs', Bhaskar told me.

Every site needed to have three rooms: awaiting room, a vaccination room and an observation room. Efforts were made to have separate entries and exits and avoid criss-cross movement of the recipients of the vaccines. The availability of adequate shaded space and safe drinking water were included in the other selection criteria.

According to Dr Parthiban: 'The layout of vaccination centres was adjusted as per the physical structure of a building. Tents were also erected where there was limited physical infrastructure available'.

Every vaccination site was to vaccinate 100 beneficiaries per day. Vaccination sessions were planned from 9 AM to 5 PM. Good internet connectivity at the sites was ensured. In the initial phase, only health facilities were chosen as vaccination centres. Subsequently, vaccination sites in government and private buildings, called 'outreach sites', were operationalized and mobile vaccination teams were also allowed.

To take care of the special needs of the elderly and differently abled, the Government of India came up with a community-based approach for vaccination, called Near to Home COVID Vaccination Centres (NHCVCs). These centres were set up in community centres, offices of resident welfare associations (RWAs), housing complexes, panchayat offices, school buildings, hostels and old age homes.[10]

Chesta Yadav deployed Delhi Transport Corporation buses for villagers to bring them to the nearest vaccination centres. She told me: 'The district machinery worked in close collaboration with RWAs in urban areas. RWA offices were used as registration centres for the non-computer-friendly citizens'. 'Anganwadi centres and Saheli Samanvay Kendras (SSKs) were made into full-time vaccination camps for better coverage', said Dr Devansh.

MOBILIZATION OF MANPOWER

The availability of skilled health workers and supporting staff was another challenge. India's UIP is powered by 1.2 million doctors and 3.07 million nurses.[2] However, aside routine immunization, they were overburdened and stressed by the pandemic.

According to Dr Manohar Agnani, the states were advised to explore avenues for the utilization of the services of medical interns, final-year MBBS students and final-year postgraduate students. They were also advised to utilize the services of final-year BSc (nursing) students under appropriate guidance.[10]

Rajesh Bhushan added: 'Human resource availability was augmented by identification and training of vaccinators from tertiary hospitals, health structures under various other departments and private sector hospitals'. He added that the existing human resources were also repurposed to suit the changing needs of health facilities.

To bridge the gap, 239,000 auxiliary nurses and midwives (ANMs) were trained to administer vaccines.[13] Rules were amended to authorize allied health workers, including 0.8 million pharmacists, to administer vaccines, subject to training and certification. Retired health workers were also deputed. States were provided with the requisite financial support under NHM and the India COVID-19 Emergency Response and Health Systems Preparedness Package for this purpose.

Akhil Arora told me that large numbers of ANMs were recruited immediately and trained. 'In addition, 25,000 community health assistants (CHAs) and 1,000 community health consultants were immediately appointed to serve the dual purpose of COVID-19 prevention and to support the vaccination drive', he added.

Apart from vaccinators, every vaccination site needed supporting manpower for verification of the recipients of vaccination shots, crowd management and overall coordination. They were drawn from different government departments.

Five people were deployed at each vaccination site. Vaccination Officer 1 pre-checked the registration status and photo identity of the recipients of the vaccine; Vaccination Officer 2 verified documents in the CoWIN system and Vaccination Officers 3 and 4 managed the crowd, monitored AEFIs and guided non-registered people. The Vaccinator Officer in each team vaccinated people. A supervisor was deployed for three to five vaccination teams.

States sourced people to form vaccination teams from wherever they could find them. 'We had sufficient vaccinators in Andhra Pradesh. However, for management of vaccination centres, we used Mahila Police (policewomen), ward and village secretariat volunteers, and Data Entry Operators in vaccination teams', Bhaskar told me.

The teams were supported by mobilizers, including accredited social health activists (ASHAs), anganwadi workers, members of village health sanitation and nutrition committees and urban local body staff. According to Akhil Arora, 'Different cadres from departments such as education, the police and Integrated Child Development Services were engaged and trained on the implementation and management aspects of COVID vaccination. A backup plan was also prepared to manage any unforeseen situation'.

TRAINING AND CAPACITY-BUILDING

Capacity-building of human resources for administration of the COVID-19 vaccine was a mammoth task considering the huge number of personnel to be trained. A critical success factor for the COVID-19 vaccination campaign was the quality of training given to vaccinators and other members of the teams deployed at the vaccination centres. Training for vaccination teams was organized in a cascade mode, leveraging innovative training channels and modalities.

While talking to me, Rajesh Bhushan elaborated on the Government of India's training strategy: 'Training was planned and conducted in a cascading manner, starting from training of trainers at the national level to the vaccination teams and the front-line health workers at the sub-district level'.

In view of the pandemic, while only the online training mode was used at the national and state levels, a mix of physical and virtual methods were used at the district and sub-district levels. Online platforms such as WebEx, Microsoft Teams, Google and the government, as well as the development partners' online training facilities, were used.

'Since the private sector was also involved in the vaccination drive, private sector personnel were trained on operationalization of the vaccination programme, and storage and recording of the COVID vaccines', Rajesh Bhushan added.

A tailored version of Integrated Government Online Training (the iGOT) portal on Digital Infrastructure for Knowledge Sharing was also used for training. The teams were trained on vaccine safety, vaccine logistics management, monitoring and supervision, management of AEFI, effective communication and use of CoWIN.

Bhaskar told me that Andhra Pradesh started with a two-day state-level workshop followed by training of all medical officers. 'Training was conducted on COVID-19 vaccine cold chain maintenance, safe injection practices and management of AEFI', he added.

'We attended the training through video conference. It was about everything from cold chain handling to management of AEFI', said Dr Mohit Rathod, Medical Officer in Charge of the Community Health Centre at Ghogla in Diu.

Apart from administration of vaccines and management of vaccination centres, people also needed training to operate the CoWIN portal. 'We trained many people in operating the CoWIN portal to address the difficulties faced by them in using its different features', said Dr V. K. Das, Director, Medical and Health Services, Dadra and Nagar Haveli and Daman and Diu.

DRY RUNS TO CHECK PREPAREDNESS

Before initiating the drive, multiple rounds of dry runs were carried out in December 2020 to identify and iron out last-minute hitches.[2,3] All major steps for the COVID-19 vaccination procedure were tested and the methods and skills learnt were rehearsed. The dry runs also assessed the operational feasibility of using the CoWIN application. Task forces at various levels reviewed observations of dry runs to take corrective measures.

Rajesh Bhushan spoke to me at length about the dry runs: 'The dry runs were conducted to field test the entire operational planning and IT platform. It was first done in four states—Andhra Pradesh, Assam, Punjab and Gujarat—on 28 and 29 December 2020, followed by an end-to-end dry run of the vaccination drives in all states and union territories at a total of 286 session sites spread across 125 districts'.

Each district conducted a dry run at three sites or more to test the mechanisms required for rollout of the COVID-19 vaccination programme and to familiarize state, district, block and hospital level officers with all aspects of the COVID-19 vaccination procedure. Dry runs included the operational processes and their linkages with the CoWIN software.

Successively, as a simulation of the actual execution, another round of dry runs in all the districts was conducted on 8 January 2021. It aimed to ensure efficient planning and management of vaccine delivery. 'Each district identified three types of session sites, including a public health facility, a private health facility and a rural or urban outreach site', said Rajesh Bhushan.

The state and union territory officers were guided in the conduct of activities for the dry run. Dr Parthiban said: 'The entire planning of the vaccination drive, including beneficiary registration, microplanning and vaccination at the planned session site, was tested under the leadership of the district magistrate'. According to Mayur Dikshit: 'This activity helped us strengthen the linkages between the planning, implementation and reporting mechanisms and identification of any residual challenges'.

COMMUNICATION AND ADVOCACY

Another vital component of the world's largest vaccination drive was an effective communication strategy to disseminate correct and timely information to the people; alleviate apprehensions, misconceptions and myths, and build confidence in the safety and efficacy of the vaccines.

A comprehensive COVID-19 vaccine communication strategy was launched on *30* December 2020 by the Ministry of Health and Family Welfare. The strategy was shared with the states. It focused on building vaccine confidence through clear, consistent and transparent messaging. The emphasis was on providing correct information on COVID-19 vaccines, addressing vaccine hesitancy and vaccine eagerness, and promoting COVID appropriate behaviour.

An orientation of state immunization and information, education and communication (IEC) officers from all the states and union territories on the COVID-19 Vaccination Communication Strategy was conducted. Rajesh Bhushan told me that the Ministry prepared IEC material and prototypes for all media—print, social and electronic media—and shared these with the states and union territories for their suitable adaptation. 'There was close coordination with 13 line ministries to disseminate the right messages through their platforms and use the structures under them to carry out vaccination and mobilization activities', he added.

Influencers such as political leaders, public health experts, doctors and government officials were roped in to endorse the safety and efficacy of vaccines. Community mobilizers and frontline workers also played a vital role. Political leaders, apart from the Prime Minister, included the union ministers and chief ministers of the states. Dr Vinod Paul, Member of the NITI Aayog; Dr Randeep

Guleria, Director, AIIMS, New Delhi, and Dr Balram Bhargava, Director General, ICMR were among the technical experts.

To promote vaccination, the Government of India roped in megastar Amitabh Bachchan. Some of the state governments also appointed brand ambassadors from the film industry. While Punjab appointed actor Sonu Sood, Maharashtra opted for actor Salman Khan to create awareness of the necessity of COVID vaccination.

A National Media Rapid Response Cell (NMRRC) was set up in New Delhi. The news and public discourse on vaccine hesitancy, vaccine eagerness and any misreporting or false information regarding the COVID-19 vaccine were closely monitored and responded to by the government. The states were also asked to do the same.

Special emphasis was placed on social media. WhatsApp, the most popular platform, was used to amplify factual information and positive messaging, and dispel rumours. A WhatsApp content toolkit, guide and content pack were developed and disseminated.

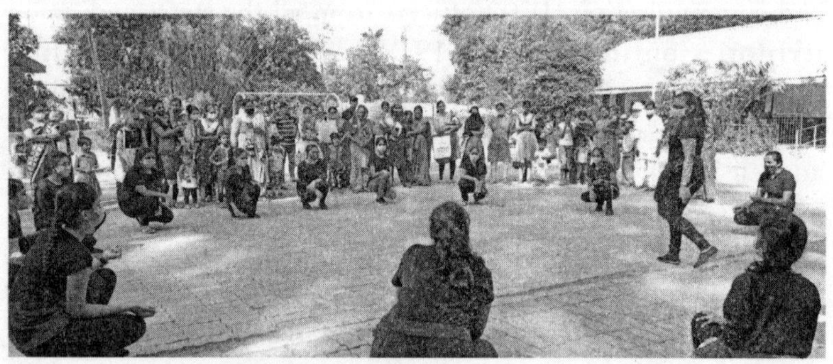

Awareness about COVID-19 Vaccination through Street Plays in Dadra and Nagar Haveli

'Sensitization of the public was initiated way before the actual commencement of the drive through pamphlets, banners, street plays, IEC *raths* and social media', Dr Muthamma said. According to Akhil Arora in Rajasthan, apart from developing attractive IEC material, the state very effectively utilized the village panchayats and CHAs to reach every person.

TV channels and radio jockeys were oriented, and op-eds by identified experts were published. Fact-check videos by key experts were also disseminated among the public. Since the global community was eagerly watching India's vaccination drive, international media was also engaged in propagating correct information and pre-empting and countering negative or false news.

VACCINE PROCUREMENT

Securing adequate supply of vaccines was the most formidable challenge. Assuming a two-dose regimen, nearly two billion doses were needed to vaccinate the entire Indian population above 18 years of age. In its budget of 2021–2022, the Government of India had allocated a sum of ₹35 billion for COVID-19 vaccinations.

On 3 January 2021, the Indian regulator granted permission for two homegrown COVID-19 vaccines, Covishield and Covaxin, for restricted use in emergency situations. On 10 January 2021, the central government placed its first purchase order.[14]

In April 2021, the government waived the requirement for bridging trials in India to expand its basket of vaccines. Bridging trials are localized clinical trials that are conducted to assess the efficacy of a vaccine in participants from a particular country. This is important because vaccines and other pharmaceuticals react differently in people with an Indian genetic makeup.

Following this, Dr Reddy's Laboratories was granted permission to import Russia-made vaccine Sputnik V. Another company was also given permission to manufacture this vaccine by using ready-to-fill bulk. Cipla Limited received the government's permission to import the Moderna vaccine from the USA.

The government also took steps to augment the domestic manufacturing capacity. These included advance payments for vaccine procurement to the SII and Bharat Biotech. The government also pre-ordered 300 million doses of another vaccine from the Indian company, Biological E. The funds provided were used by these manufacturers to augment their capacity.

Financial support was provided to domestic manufacturers under 'Mission COVID Suraksha'. Three government enterprises, Indian Immunologicals Ltd, Bharat Immunologicals Ltd and Haffkine Institute, were transferred the technology to manufacture Covaxin.[15]

However, the price caps set by the Indian government, a lack of critical raw materials and a fire that damaged a part of SII's facility got in the way of ramping up vaccine production.[16]

PRIORITIZATION OF VACCINE RECIPIENTS

India had planned a phased rollout of vaccination, keeping in view its huge population, constraints on vaccine supplies, manpower, and infrastructure, and the evolving nature of the pandemic.[17] 'Learning from global best practices, policy-related decisions and strategic guidance for rollout of the vaccination programme in phases was guided by the NEGVAC,' said Rajesh Bhushan.

Prioritization of beneficiaries was undertaken to utilize the available COVID-19 vaccines in such a manner as to maximize the impact in terms of protection of the COVID-19 response system, and reduction of mortality and morbidity associated with COVID-19. This brought to the fore healthcare and frontline workers and elderly people with comorbidities. An analysis of COVID-19-related mortality revealed that people over 60 years of age and those between 45 and 59 years of age with comorbidities, such as diabetes, hypertension and cardiovascular and respiratory diseases contributed to a large majority of deaths.[11,18]

Based on the guidance from the NEGVAC, India commenced its vaccination drive with high-risk groups: healthcare providers and workers in healthcare settings. This was followed by frontline workers, which included police personnel. As a lack of availability of vaccines eased, other groups were included on the recommendation of the NEGVAC, based on scientific evidence and global practices.

After health and frontline workers, people over the age of 60 and those between 45 and 59 years of age with specific comorbidities were selected for vaccination. After this, the drive included everyone over the age of 45, followed by all people over 18 years of age. Vaccination of children commenced from 3 January 2022 for children in the age group of 15 to 18 years followed by the children in the 12 to 14 years age from 16 March 2022.

FIRST PHASE: PROTECTING HEALTH AND FRONTLINE WORKERS

India launched its National COVID-19 Vaccination Programme on 16 January 2021. 'Today marks the beginning of a long and decisive phase in India's fight against the pandemic,' Prime Minister Modi said while launching the drive. The atmosphere was festive. In many places, the COVID-19 vaccine was welcomed with bands, flowers, firecrackers and *puja*.

The first phase of the programme aimed at inoculating 30 million healthcare and frontline Corona workers. Manish Kumar, a 34-year-old sanitation worker at Delhi's AIIMS, became the first person in India to receive the vaccination. And despite apprehensions, almost 200,000 workers got themselves vaccinated on the first day of the vaccine rollout.

India inoculated 3 million people in the first 15 days. The USA took 18 days and the United Kingdom 36 days to achieve this feat. As many as 8.4 million people were vaccinated in the first month.

Vaccination of 20 million frontline workers (FLWs) started on 2 February 2021, with 100 per cent of the vaccines being procured by the Government of India and provided free of cost to state governments.

A digital vaccination certificate with details was provided to the vaccinated person after the vaccination. They were then monitored for 30 minutes to check for any adverse reactions.

SECOND PHASE: PROTECTING THE VULNERABLE

As systems and processes stabilized, the immunization campaign was expanded from 1 March 2021. This phase aimed at protecting 270 million people who were considered part of the most vulnerable section of the population. This included people aged 60 years or older and those aged 45 years or older who had any of the 20 specified comorbidities. Advanced self-registration and appointments were made available to citizens through the CoWIN Portal. Prime Minister Modi was administered the vaccine on the first day of this phase. He preferred the indigenously developed Covaxin.

Initially, vaccination centres were in government health facilities only. Subsequently, private hospitals were also enlisted at the prescribed rate of ₹250 per dose.

To begin with, vaccines were only administered to pre-registered beneficiaries as per their allotted date and time. However, taking into account the initial low turnout, walk-in vaccinations were allowed from the second week.[7]

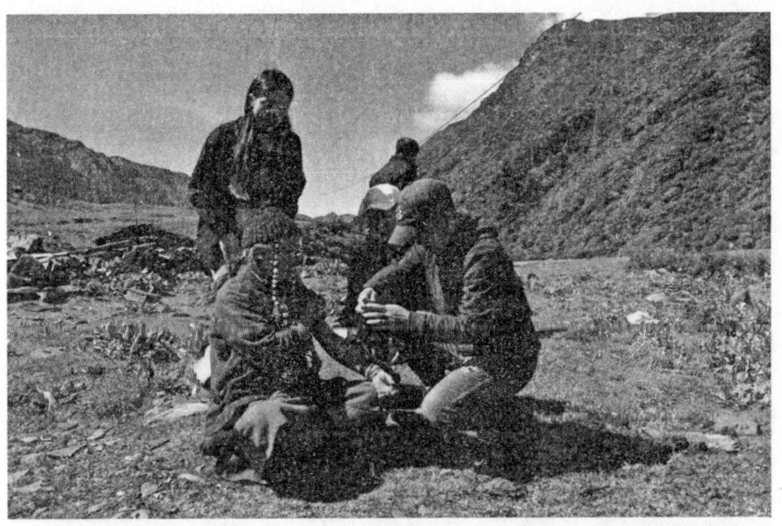

A Shepherd Family being Vaccinated in a Remote Area of Arunachal Pradesh

THIRD PHASE: OVERCOMING VACCINE RELUCTANCE

The third phase of COVID-19 vaccination drive began on 1 April 2021 All persons above 45 years of age were made eligible for inoculation.

However, the initial enthusiasm of people had waned by then. Questions about the efficacy and safety of vaccines had made people suspicious. The distance from vaccination centres, technical glitches in Co-WIN, fever after vaccination and consequent wage loss, and requirement of a doctor's certificate regarding the health problems of persons between 45 and 59 years of age also muted people's enthusiasm to take vaccines. The steady decline in cases for months also led to vaccine indifference.[19]

To accelerate the drive, walk-in vaccinations were started and new vaccination centres were set up. Some states set up counselling centres to dissipate fears about vaccines.[20] The government also introduced its NHCVC scheme and immunization at workplace.

Vaccination teams made heroic efforts to reach inaccessible areas and reluctant people. Special teams in Jammu and Kashmir travelled for hours on foot and horseback to reach the remote villages of Gujjars and Bakarwals who migrate to the mountains of Kashmir in summer. The deputy commissioner of the Tawang district in Arunachal Pradesh trekked for nine hours to reach Brokpas, the yak herders who live at a height of 14,000 feet.

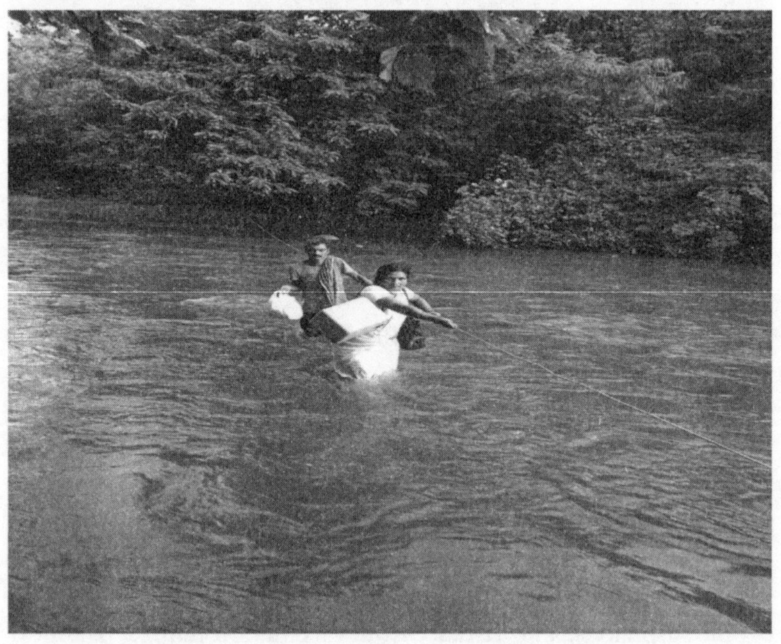

A Frontline Worker in Andhra Pradesh on COVID-19 Vaccination Mission

An all-women team in Meghalaya trekked for hours through hills, amidst rain and slush in an area infested with leeches and snakes to take the vaccines to far-flung villages.

Health staff carried vaccine vials on their bikes and scooters and inoculated people in agricultural farms, ration shops, temples, under roadside trees, inside buses, at wedding sites and wherever they found eligible people.[21,22]

The Prime Minister Modi proposed a four-day concerted campaign, 'Teeka Utsav' (vaccination festival) from 11 April 2021 to give a boost to the vaccination drive. More than 10 million people were vaccinated during the Teeka Utsav.

FOURTH PHASE: BATTLING SCARCITY

A new challenge, scarcity of vaccines, was slowly emerging. During April and May 2021, there was a steep rise in the number of COVID-19 cases in India. From 80,000 cases on 1 April 2021, it soared to 414,000 cases on 6 May 2021. This was the highest ever single-day record globally. The death toll climbed in tandem and hit 6,148 on 9 June 2021. The resurgence of cases drove people to vaccination centres.

This led to a rethinking within the government of its vaccination strategy. It announced a Liberalised Pricing and Accelerated National COVID-19 Vaccination Strategy on 19 April 2021, which became effective from 1 May 2021. This strategy opened up vaccination for everyone over the age of 18.

The Centre also conceded to the demand of the states to allow them to procure and administer vaccines as per their own prioritization. The new policy aimed at incentivizing vaccine manufacturers to produce more vaccines by providing them with a window to charge a higher rate from states and private hospitals.

The new strategy converted the vaccination drive into a mixed-mode operation. The Centre provided vaccines to the states for free vaccination of healthcare workers, frontline workers and the 45-plus people. The state governments were assigned the responsibility of procuring and vaccinating the 18–44 age group.[23]

The manufacturers were asked to supply 50 per cent of the monthly quota of vaccines released by the CDL to the central government and the rest to the state governments and private hospitals at pre-declared prices. Imported vaccines were not procured by the

Indian Government. But private hospitals, corporates and other non-government entities were allowed to procure and use them.

The new policy made an additional 940 million people eligible for vaccination overnight. However, the vaccine supply did not increase in tandem with the eligibility criteria.[19]

States could not procure vaccine doses from Indian manufacturers in sufficient quantities. Their procurement efforts in the international market failed as well. Therefore, things soon began to go awry. Everyone, including those over 45 years old, was finding it difficult to get vaccinated.

Due to the dwindling supply, the daily average of vaccines administered in May 2021 declined to 1.8 million doses from 3.65 million doses administered from 1 April to 10 April 2021.

Critics blamed the situation on poor planning, piecemeal procurement of vaccines, late pre-ordering of vaccines, and a vaccination policy that was unmindful of supplies. The Indian government's vaccine diplomacy was also accused of contributing to the shortage.

Another failure pointed out by critics was non-listing of India's huge manufacturing capabilities that could have been repurposed into vaccine production lines. The government's initiative to provide financial support and rights to four companies to manufacture Covaxin was also criticized as one that came too late.

FASTEST FINGER FIRST

Due to the shortfall in supply, booking a slot for vaccination online had become a challenging task. Some people complained that it was akin to playing the game 'fastest finger first' on the popular TV show *Kaun Banega Crore Pati*.

Sneha, one of the recipients of the vaccine, told me that it took her half a day to book an appointment online for a COVID-19 vaccination and about how slots were getting filled up in three seconds.

'Extreme vaccine eagerness was witnessed with the initiation of vaccination in the age group of 18 to 45 years', said Akhil Arora during the interview. 'Crowding at CVCs was observed due to the surge of people from nearby states', Dr Muthamma told us. 'We had to deploy police during this period', said Bhaskar. Dr Parthiban also recalled the challenges faced during this phase.

CoWIN came under tremendous stress. People were stuck in an OTP loop for hours. On Twitter, the hashtag #WaitingForOTP trended, followed by memes and jokes. Some tech-savvy youngsters even resorted to writing codes to corner elusive appointments.

THE U TURN

The new liberalized policy could not be sustained for long. Many states voiced their difficulties in managing the funding, procurement and logistics of vaccines. Small private hospitals reported difficulties in securing vaccines.

It is at this point that the vaccination policy saw a reversal. The central government decided to take over the reins of the inoculation exercise from 21 June 2021.

As per the new guidelines, the Government of India started procuring 75 per cent of the vaccines that were manufactured in India. These were provided free of cost to states on the basis of their pro-rata target population and consumption pattern with disincentives for vaccine wastage.

PROTECTING CHILDREN AND BOOSTING IMMUNITY OF HEALTH WORKERS AND THE ELDERLY

Another phase in India's vaccination drive started with 2022 ushering in a third wave of COVID-19. On 25 December 2021, Prime Minister Modi announced that vaccination for children aged 15 years and above would commence from 3 January 2022.

It was also decided to administer a 'precaution' dose to frontline workers and people 60 years and above with comorbidities.

In this segment, over 150,000 children, 77,000 health workers and 100,000 senior citizens with co-morbidities had been vaccinated by 15 January 2022.[2]

MILESTONES ACHIEVED AND CHALLENGES AHEAD

In its COVID-19 vaccination drive, India saw a series of milestones. As per the CoWIN dashboard, the #SabkoVaccineMuftVaccine movement saw the country marching ahead of the one billion mark with delivery of 1,861,862,924 vaccinations by 13 April 2022. Moreover, 841,301,909 people had been fully vaccinated by then.[24,25]

A perceptible acceleration in the pace of vaccination was witnessed with time. While it took 85 days to administer the first 100 million doses, the next 10 million were administered in 45 days, 29 days, 24 days and 20 days.[25] Thereafter, India took just 76 days to jump from 500 million to one billion, and another 75 days to cross the 1.5 billion mark. During the journey, India set a world record of more than 25 million vaccinations in a day on 17 September 2020, on the occasion of the birthday of Prime Minister Modi. The country's inoculation drive has become the world's largest in terms of the daily vaccinations being administered as well as total shots being given.[24]

On 16 January 2022, India completed a year of administering vaccination to its citizens against COVID-19. The day was marked by the launch of a postal stamp on India's feat in developing an indigenous COVID-19 vaccine. The country had administered 1,572,229,080 vaccine doses and 656,773,758 people had received both the shots. Out of the total doses, males received 799,896,134 shots and females 763,462,966.[24]

However, India has a long way to go before its citizens can achieve a mask-free life again. Since the immunity provided by the vaccines is expected to last for only a year, India has to not only complete administering two doses to eligible people, but also to arrange booster doses for them.

MONITORING ADVERSE EVENTS

An Adverse Event Following Immunization (AEFI) is any untoward medical occurrence following immunization that is not necessarily caused by the vaccine. AEFIs are classified as minor, severe and serious. Minor AEFI includes common self-limiting reactions such as swelling at the injection site, pain, fever, irritability and malaise. Severe AEFI can be disabling but rarely life-threatening, for instance, anaphylaxis and high fever. Serious AEFI requires in-patient hospitalization and may result in significant disability and also death.

In view of limited safety data on COVID-19 vaccines, it was important to monitor AEFI and better understand the safety profile of the vaccines. It is also important to gain the confidence of people and prevent fear-mongering about vaccines. Efforts have been made to prevent AEFI due to immunization errors through proper training.

In CoWIN's beneficiary module, provision has been made for reporting AEFIs. It is mandated that all adverse events must be reported. Vaccinators and supervisors have been tasked with providing primary treatment of all AEFIs. Cases requiring more specialized care are referred to the nearest health facility.

However, the number of AEFIs reported was low and most of them were classified as 'minor'. By 14 April 2022, their proportion was 0.005 per cent.[24]

VACCINE POLITICS

The COVID-19 vaccination drive witnessed hectic political discussion. When vaccination began, some political leaders tried to discredit the vaccines by saying that people were being treated like rats and guinea pigs by administering vaccines to those who had not completed the mandatory trials.[26] The opposition also attacked the government over the 'Thank You Modi Ji' campaign on the 'free vaccination drive' as well as the Prime Minister's picture being on vaccination certificates.

The Government's focus then shifted to the demand for providing vaccines free of cost to everyone. Over-reliance on CoWIN to administer vaccines was also criticized as being biased against the poor and rural citizens.

The next political 'slugfest' was witnessed when vaccination was opened to everyone. Many states were critical of the central government's prioritized approach and demanded their freedom to procure and administer vaccines.

When the government conceded to their demand, its political opponents criticized the policy as being 'not well thought out' and a 'clever political ploy' rather than a solution. The policy was also criticized for making it a 'seller's market', for opening up 'debilitating competition among states' and for triggering a 'desperate free-for-all rush' to secure jabs. The Centre was accused of abdicating its responsibility and passing the buck to the states.

The central government, on the other hand, contended that the new policy had made pricing, procurement, eligibility and administration of vaccines flexible and open.

After much political posturing, the states went back to the Centre requesting it to supply vaccines. The Prime Minister Modi conceded to their demand. 'Whether it's the poor, the lower middle class, the middle class or the upper-middle class, under the central government's programme, everyone will get free vaccines', he had said in his address to the nation.

Any mass vaccination drive needs to overcome many formidable challenges to be successful. These challenges are posed by both hesitancy and eagerness to get vaccinated. Fair and equitable availability of vaccines are other formidable challenges. The next chapter is dedicated to these critical aspects of the fight against infectious diseases.

REFERENCES

1. The BMJ. India's challenges with Covid-19 vaccination [online]. The BMJ. 2021. Available from: https://blogs.bmj.com/bmj/2021/06/03/indias-challenges-with-covid-19-vaccination/
2. Kapur K. India's historic vaccination drive: Evaluating the stakes, hurdles and opportunities [online]. ORF. 2021. Available from: https://www.orfonline.org/research/india-historic-vaccination-drive-evaluating-stakes-hurdles opportunities/#_ednref5
3. Sharma P, Pardeshi G. Rollout of COVID-19 vaccination in India: A SWOT analysis. Disaster Medicine and Public Health Preparedness. 6 April 2021. 1–4.
4. Bhatia V. Explained: What is eVIN, and how will it be used for distributing Covid-19 vaccines? [Internet]. *The Indian Express*. 2020 [cited 16 January 2022]. Available from: https://indianexpress.com/article/explained/what-is-evin-and-how-will-it-be-used-for-distributing-covid-19-vaccine-7065083/
5. Electronic Vaccine Intelligence Network (eVIN) [Internet]. Nhp.gov.in. 2021 [cited 16 January 2022]. Available from: https://www.nhp.gov.in/electronic-vaccine-intelligence-network(evin)_pg/
6. ET Bureau. India has done well in development of vaccines: Health Minister Harsh Vardhan [Internet]. *The Economic Times*. 2021 [cited 16 January 2022]. Available from: https://economictimes.indiatimes.com/industry/healthcare/biotech/healthcare/india-has-done-well-in-the-development-of-vaccines-health-minister-harsh-vardhan/articleshow/80174116.cms?utm_source=contentofinterest&utm_medium=text&utm_campaign=cppst
7. Srivastava RK, Ish P. COVID. The initial experience of COVID-19 vaccination from a tertiary care centre in India. Monaldi Archives for Chest Disease. 31 March 2021.
8. *Times of India* [Internet]. Covid-19: India vaccinates 54.7% healthcare workers registered on CoWin platform. Accessed: 22 February 2021. Available from: https://timesofindia.indiatimes.com/india/covid-19-india-vaccinates-54-7-healthcareworkers-registered-on-cowin-platform/articleshow/80725869.cms
9. Mohfw.gov.in. 2020. Guidance note for COWIN 2.0. [online] Available from: https://www.mohfw.gov.in/pdf/GuidancedocCOWIN2.pdf[Accessed 7 August 2021].

10. Centre Affidavit. Vaccine Policy in Supreme Court in Civil Writ 3 of 2021 [Internet]. Livelaw.in. 2021 [cited 16 January 2022]. Available from: https://www.livelaw.in/pdf_upload/centre-affidavit-vaccine-policy-395568.pdf
11. Leroy Leo and Goutam Das, 'Is India Ready to Deliver a Vaccine to a Billion People?' LiveMint, 12 October 2020.
12. Brendan Borrell. The tree that could help stop the pandemic. The Atlantic, 21 October 2020, https://www.theatlantic.com/science/archive/2020/10/single-tree-species-may-hold-key-coronavirus-vaccine/616792/
13. Kumar V M, S R Pandi-Perumal, I Trakht, S P Thyagarajan. Strategy for COVID-19 vaccination in India: the country with the second-highest population and number of cases. *NPJ Vaccines*. 2021 April;6(1):1–7.
14. Bagcchi S. The world's largest COVID-19 vaccination campaign. *The Lancet Infectious Diseases*. 2021 March;(3):323.
15. Naik S. et al. A COVID-19 Vaccine deployment strategy for India. *Indian Public Policy Review*. 2020;1(2): 42–58.
16. NPR.org. 2021. India is the world's biggest vaccine maker. Yet only 4% of Indians are vaccinated. [online] Available from: https://www.npr.org/sections/goatsandsoda/2021/06/29/1011022472/india-is-the-worlds-biggest-vaccine-maker-yet-only-4-of-indians-are-vaccinated[Accessed 11 August 2021].
17. COVID-19 vaccines operational guidelines [Internet]. Main.mohfw.gov.in. 2020 [cited 2 August 2021]. Available from: https://main.mohfw.gov.in/sites/default/files/COVID19VaccineOG111Chapter16.pdf
18. Updates on COVID-19. Ministry of Health and Family Welfare, June 2020. https://pib.gov.in/PressReleasePage.aspx?PRID=1628696
19. Pandey A, Sah P, Moghadas SM, Mandal S, Banerjee S, Hotez PJ, Galvani AP. Challenges facing COVID-19 vaccination in India: Lessons from the initial vaccine rollout. *Journal of Global Health*. 2021;11.
20. *Time*. 2021. India's vaccine rollout stumbles as COVID-19 cases decline. That's bad news for the rest of the world. [online] Available from: https://time.com/5940963/india-covid-19-vaccine-rollout/[Accessed 11 August 2021].
21. *Times of India*. 2021. Karnataka: In Yadgir, officials jab people in farms, PDS shops | Bengaluru News. *Times of India*. [online] Available from: https://timesofindia.indiatimes.com/city/bengaluru/karnataka-in-yadgir-officials-jab-people-in-farms-pds-shops/articleshow/83942925.cms[Accessed 9 August 2021].
22. Who.int. 2021. WHO support in India. [online] Available from: https://www.who.int/india/who-support-in-india[Accessed 12 August 2021].
23. Revised guidelines for implementation of national COVID vaccination program [Internet]. Mohfw.gov.in. 2021 [cited 2 August 2021]. Available from: https://www.mohfw.gov.in/pdf/RevisedVaccinationGuidelines.pdf
24. CoWIN Dashboard [Internet]. Dashboard.cowin.gov.in. 2022 [cited 17 January 2022]. Available from: https://dashboard.cowin.gov.in/

25. Outlook Web Desk. 100 Crore Shots: How India Achieved Covid-19 Vaccination Milestone In 280 Days [Internet]. 2021 [cited 17 January 2022]. Available from: https://www.outlookindia.com/website/story/india-news-one-billion-club-how-india-crossed-the-covid-19-vaccine-milestone-in-279-days/398384
26. How BJP is turning India's COVID vaccine drive into a political campaign [Internet]. *The Wire*. 2021 [cited 5 September 2021]. Available from: https://thewire.in/politics/bjp-narendra-modi-covid-19-vaccine-pr-drive

Chapter 7

Tackling Vaccine Hesitancy, Equity and Eagerness

From smallpox to COVID-19, vaccines have time and time again proved their worth as the most potent weapons to decimate infectious diseases. However, inoculation drives have faced the complex challenges of vaccine hesitancy, equity and, interestingly, eagerness.

VACCINE HESITANCY: A COMPLEX AND PERVASIVE CHALLENGE

Vaccine hesitancy is the delay in acceptance, reluctance or refusal of vaccination.[1] It's ubiquitous and has been recognized as one of the top 10 threats to global health.[2] Vaccine hesitancy creates pockets of sub-optimal vaccine coverage, increasing the risk of vaccine-preventable diseases (VPDs).[3,4]

Vaccine hesitancy is complex and multidimensional. It varies across time, places and vaccines.[5,6] According to 'the 5C model', five different levels of the determinants of vaccine hesitancy include confidence, complacency, constraints or convenience, risk calculation and collective responsibility.[7] The WHO has come up with its '3C model' of vaccine hesitancy: complacency, convenience and confidence.[8]

Confidence is people's trust in government policies, health systems, healthcare providers, and the effectiveness and safety of vaccines. Complacency emanates from the reduced risk perception of

VPDs. Convenience encompasses acceptability, affordability and availability of vaccines.

The determinants of vaccination-related decisions can be contextual, individual or organizational. Gender, religion and politics are contextual determinants, as are cultural and historical factors, vaccine communication, social norms and societal pressure. Individual determinants include emotions, values, family or community members' experiences with vaccines, as well as education, awareness, knowledge, trust, and the perceived risks and benefits of immunization. Organizational determinants include administration of vaccines and processes such as the design, mode and schedule of immunization, as well as overall communication and adequate supplies.[9,10]

Vaccine hesitancy is steadily rising and has become a global phenomenon due to the technological revolution. Understanding its complexity is critical in strategizing efforts to enhance vaccine uptake.

But is vaccine hesitancy an entirely new phenomenon?

ANTI-VEXERS: AS OLD AS VACCINES

The anti-vaccine movement was born with the discovery of the first vaccine by Edward Jenner in 1796.[11] While Jenner was lauded for his discovery, he was also accused of bestiality. The clergy called vaccination 'unchristian'. Some people considered vaccines to be 'poisonous, filthy, loathsome and damnable stuff', which caused 'corruption of the blood'.[3]

Jenner's critics even tried to scare people by saying that the recipients of the vaccines would develop bovine features. British satirist James Gillray published a cartoon in 1802 that showed cows emerging from different parts of the bodies of persons inoculated with cowpox vaccine.[9]

Anti-vaxxers started organizing like-minded people, including medical practitioners, against vaccines.[3] Their safety concerns were genuine, however, since the smallpox vaccine was made from pus and its chances of contamination with tetanus bacillus were high.[12]

COMPULSORY VACCINATION STIRS PROTESTS

In the mid-19th century, smallpox vaccination was made compulsory in many countries. This was considered an attack on personal liberty and was strongly contested. Numerous anti-vaccination leagues, tracts, journals and books appeared.[13] Public health authorities faced court battles, pamphlet wars and there were riots too.[12]

In the USA, the matter went up to the Supreme Court in a case titled 'Jacobson v. Massachusetts'. Although the court upheld the government's authority to mandate vaccination, the issue remained a source of tension between the health authorities and the public.

Aggrieved parents initiated an anti-vaccination campaign with the slogan 'Reject Big Pharma'. Concerns about profiteering by vaccine manufacturers, voiced then, undermine vaccine confidence even today.

In Montréal, the campaign was led by a physician called Dr Alexander Ross. He was the editor of *The Anti-vaccinator*. He publicized conspiracy theories, and exaggerated the vaccine contamination risk and the issue of personal liberties. He said the vaccinated were 'driven like dumb animals'. But surprisingly, when the epidemic struck, he got himself vaccinated quietly.[14]

New and highly effective vaccines discovered in the 20th century witnessed public protests as well.[9,15]

ASSAULTS AND ATTEMPTS TO MURDER VACCINATORS IN INDIA

Resistance to the smallpox vaccine has been reported in India as well. From simple refusal to get vaccinated, the resistance manifested itself in violent physical assaults on vaccinators. Fear of vaccination is natural. Multiple cuts were inflicted by a sharp instrument to inoculate the lymph. Arm-to-arm vaccination was considered cruel, with children bearing pain multiple times for extraction of lymph. Some children even died from fatigue and prolonged exposure during vaccination trips.[16]

Indians also suspected that vaccination was an instrument of the British Raj. Numerous rumours and conspiracy theories were doing the rounds: children were being vaccinated so that they could be traced easily by the police, the colonists were purposely infecting locals with plague to kill them and the process was being used to harvest the blood of children.[16] These were some of the damaging rumours that surfaced about vaccination.

Indians' poverty also bred vaccine hesitancy, as vaccinators charged a fee. Religious misconceptions such as smallpox being the wrath of an Indian Goddess, the sacred nature of the cow, caste discrimination leading to fears among the upper caste populace of mixing their blood with that of lower caste people during arm-to-arm vaccination, and the ancient fear of variolation also contributed to this resistance.

WAS MAHATMA GANDHI OPPOSED TO VACCINATION?

It has been reported that Mahatma Gandhi strongly opposed vaccination when he was in South Africa in 1913. 'Vaccination is a filthy remedy. Vaccine from an infected cow is introduced into our bodies.... I personally feel that in taking this vaccine we are guilty of sacrilege', he said.[17,18]

In a letter to Manilal and Sushila Gandhi, and also in his article in *Navjivan* in 1929, Mahatma Gandhi wondered 'how vegetarians can ever take such vaccines'? He thought vaccination was 'tantamount to partaking of beef'.[17,19]

ANTI-VAXXERS PLAY WITH HUMAN LIFE

The history of vaccination is replete with the victories of anti-vaxxers, which were publicized through their propaganda and rumour mills. These triumphs eroded people's trust in vaccines, precipitated their fears and pushed inoculation rates down.

Montréal Massacre

In the early 1880s, Montréal was in the grip of vaccine hesitancy emanating from a complex cocktail of politics, social forces, misunderstanding of medical advances and deeply held beliefs.[14] Vaccination rates had plummeted.

A train arrived in Montréal from Chicago in March 1885 with the smallpox demon on board. The infected person was Geroge Longley, the train conductor. He checked-in at Hôtel-Dieu, received medical attention and recovered, but not before infecting a laundry maid called Pélagie Robichaud. She died on 2 April 1885, and soon smallpox was everywhere.

The epidemic lasted till November 1885 and killed 2 per cent of Montréal's population: 90 per cent of the dead were from the eastern part of the city where vaccine resistance was most pronounced.[14]

Anti-vaxxers: Claimed Lives in the 19th Century Europe and America

In the 19th century, an Anti-vaccination League was also formed in the USA, the United Kingdom and other European countries. Their campaigns were based on people's religious objections, and concerns about the vaccines' effectiveness and individual rights. The league in Stockholm was the most influential. Its influence led to a drop in vaccination rates in Stockholm to 40 per cent, compared to 90 per cent in the rest of the country. Then smallpox struck in 1874 and caused 4,063 fatalities.[14]

In Minnesota in the USA, Lora C. Little was an influential agitator. She published *The Liberator*, an anti-vaccine monthly. In 1918, she published a pamphlet, *Vaccination: An Egregious Failure*. Her campaign resulted in the government going back on its mandate of making smallpox vaccination compulsory before children could attend school in 1903. The smallpox epidemic struck soon and infected 28,000 children.[14]

Vaccine Tragedies

The loudest public outcries against vaccines have been historically seen due to occurrence of deaths and serious diseases in close temporal proximity to vaccination. Here are some of these.

Contaminated Bottle Cap Kills Thousands

In March 1902, 19 people died in Mulkowal village in Punjab in India after being inoculated with the plague vaccine. The inquiry commission concluded that the vaccine bottle was contaminated in the manufacturing lab. Resultant mistrust and vaccine refusal by people led to plague outbreaks killing thousands.[20]

Many years later, it was proved that the deaths were due to contamination with the tetanus bacilli at the vaccination site from the cap of a vaccine bottle that had fallen on the ground and was put back without sterilizing it.

Dark Cloud over the Reputation of the BCG Vaccine

The discovery of the BCG vaccine made from *mycobacterium bovis* to protect people against the deadly tuberculosis was a significant scientific victory. The disease was reporting 3 per cent morbidity and 20 per cent to 43 per cent mortality.[21] After the vaccine passed a series of safety and protective efficacy tests in animals, the first baby was vaccinated by Weill-Hallé in 1921 at the Hôpital de la Charité (presently the Hôtel Dieu) in Paris.[22] But tragedy struck soon.

In 1929, 252 infants were administered a locally prepared BCG vaccine in Lübeck in Germany; 72 of them died from tuberculosis and 137 contracted chronic forms of the disease. The catastrophe was a big setback for the vaccine. Two German tuberculosis experts, Bruno and Ludwing Lange, carried out investigations. They found that the BCG vaccine given to these children was accidentally contaminated by a human tubercle bacilli strain, which were being studied in the same laboratory.[21]

Cutter Incident

In April 1955, then USA reported 40,000 cases of polio in children who were administered polio vaccine manufactured by Cutter Laboratories: 260 children were left paralysed and 10 died. Investigations revealed that the process used by the company to inactivate the virus was defective. The mass vaccination programme had to be abandoned.[23]

A number of civil lawsuits were filed against the company, which had to pay huge monetary damages.

Swine Flu Fiasco

In 1976, the President of the USA, Gerald Ford, launched an immunization campaign against swine flu. Shortly after being vaccinated, three elderly people had heart attacks. Although a later analysis concluded that the heart attacks were surely coincidental, it resulted in raising the collective anxiety levels of people.

Moreover, two weeks after immunization, an untoward increase in the Guillain–Barré Syndrome (GBS), a rare neurologic disease, was reported. This was linked to the swine flu vaccine and posed a challenge to vaccination in general. The government was forced to abandon its vaccination campaign.[3]

A study conducted in 2003 concludes that the recipients of the influenza vaccine in 1976 had an increased risk of GBS. However, the exact reason for the association remains unknown.

Dengvaxia Backfires

In 2016, the Philippines embarked on a mass immunization campaign against dengue fever using the Dengvaxia vaccine. The vaccine was manufactured by the French pharmaceutical company Sanofi Pasteur. However, after two years of its launch, Sanofi announced that in people who have not had previous dengue infection, Dengvaxia may cause 'more severe disease'. By then, over 800,000 children had already been inoculated.[24]

The public attorney's office started criminal investigations, which received huge publicity. The focal point of the investigation was the deaths of many children who had been inoculated.[24]

HPV Vaccine Associated with Deaths

The HPV is the main cause of cervical cancer, the second most common cancer in Indian women. HPV vaccine stirred up a controversy in India when seven girls died after being inoculated in 2010. An inquiry committee was instituted, which concluded that the vaccines were not responsible for the deaths. However, the vaccine continues to face opposition.[25]

VACCINE-RELATED CONTROVERSIES

All through their history, vaccines have attracted scepticism and resulted in conspiracy theories. They have enhanced risk perception and eroded trust in vaccines. Let's discuss about some of them.

DTP Controversy

A report published by the Great Ormond Street Hospital for Sick Children in London in 1970 resulted in the modern-day anti-vaccination movement. It was reported that 36 children suffered serious neurological conditions following DTP vaccination. The report received significant media attention around the world.

An Association of Parents of Vaccine Damaged Children was born. DPT Vaccine uptake declined in the United Kingdom from 81 per cent to 22 per cent by 1977. This resulted in three major epidemics of pertussis, with 100,000 cases and at least 36 deaths. By the mid-1980s, the controversy had swept through most of Europe, the USA, the Soviet Union, Australia and Japan. Countries suspended their use of the whole-cell pertussis vaccine for infants. Major outbreak of pertussis followed.[3,9,26]

Vaccination Roulette

In the USA, a documentary entitled *DTP: Vaccination Roulette* stirred up a big controversy in 1982. It featured the emotional profiles of children believed by their parents to have been harmed by the DPT vaccine. It was alleged that the pertussis component of the DTP vaccine caused severe brain damage, mental retardation and seizures in children.

Concerned and angry parents formed the victim advocacy group 'Dissatisfied Parents Together'. They accused the government of regulatory malfeasance or indifference. Many lawsuits were also filed against leading vaccine manufacturers.[3] The US Congress responded by passing the National Childhood Vaccine Injury Bill in 1988 to protect manufacturers from lawsuits through the Vaccine Injury Compensation Program.

Although the claims were eventually disproved, the damage had been done. It was clear that the vaccine unmasks rather than causes infantile spasms.

Carcinogenic Polio Vaccine

In 1960, American researcher Bernice Eddy reported the development of tumours in hamsters injected with the monkey kidney mixture on which polio vaccine was bred. Further investigations revealed that the polio vaccine was contaminated with monkey virus SV40. However, follow-up studies found that SV40 does not cause cancer in humans.

However, in mid-1990, Dr Michele Carbone and his colleagues detected SV40 DNA in human tumours by using molecular techniques. People sued SV40-contaminated polio vaccine manufacturers for their negligence. However, SV40 was detected in human tumours in some laboratories and not in others. Therefore, it was believed that the presence of SV40 in various tumours may be due to contamination in laboratories.

Wakefield Effect

British physician Dr Andrew Wakefield whipped a global hysteria among parents in 1998. In a study published in the *Lancet*, he claimed that MMR vaccination caused ASDs in children. His findings were lapped up by anti-vaxxers and added fire to the flame.

Complaints poured in, leading to setting up of the Omnibus Autism Proceeding to examine the causal link. However, no link could be found. It was later revealed that Dr Wakefield committed fraud, was being paid by a personal injury lawyer and intentionally altered his findings. The *Lancet* retracted the study in 2010. Dr Wakefield was stripped of his medical license. However, this had repercussions on people's compliance with mandates relating to the MMR vaccine for several years and led to numerous epidemics.[11]

Does Vaccine Cause Multiple Sclerosis and Narcolepsy ?

In 1998, researchers raised concerns in France that hepatitis B vaccination may be linked with the development of multiple sclerosis, a progressive nerve disease. Subsequently, a large body of research found no link between the two.[15,27]

Finland and some other European countries reported increased risk of narcolepsy, a chronic sleep disorder, following inoculation of a monovalent H1N1 influenza vaccine. However, no such link could be detected in future studies.

MYTHS, MISINFORMATION AND RUMOURS

'Vaccinophobia' is spurred by myths and misinformation about vaccines.[28] The internet and social media have brought crushing waves of vaccine misinformation to parents during COVID-19. Unproven vaccine safety scares, seeds doubt and distrusts and breeds rumours.[29]

HOW MANY PRICKS CAN A CHILD'S BODY TAKE?

Parents have been misinformed about the multiple inoculations administered to children in the first two years of their lives. They were told that they overwhelm or weaken an immature immune system. However, there is no association between the number of antigens administered and any neuropsychological disorders found.[3,29]

In early life, a child is exposed to many infections. Therefore, it is important that protection against them is built. Multiple inoculations at the same time have been found to be safe, immunologically effective and logistically and economically efficient.[30,31]

PRESERVATIVE PROPAGATES ASDS

Vaccination foes thrive on creating a fear psychosis. They claim that vaccines do not work well and contain harmful ingredients. Anti-vaxxers tried to link thimerosal, a mercury-containing anti-fungal preservative used in vaccines with increased risk of neurodevelopmental disorders.[29] However, thimerosal contains ethyl-mercury, which is disintegrated and excreted rapidly and is thus less likely to accumulate in the body and cause harm.

A large number of studies conducted on the subject have found no link between thimerosal-containing vaccines and autism or other developmental disabilities. Nonetheless, as a precautionary measure, countries have shifted to thimerosal free childhood vaccines.[29]

VACCINES: STERILIZATION WEAPONS

Rumours that vaccines cause infertility and are administered to sterilize people do the rounds across countries. In Cameroon, rumours that childhood vaccines are being administered to sterilize women had thwarted the country's immunization campaign in 1990. Similarly, sterlization rumours about tetanus vaccination had halted the campaign in Philippines in the 1990s.

The polio vaccination drive in Nigeria failed in 2003 due to sterilization-related rumours.[9] Fear of infertility due to the polio vaccine was found to be pronounced in Pakistan and Afghanistan, and is one of the reasons why the countries are still not polio free.[25]

VACCINES NOT HALAL

There are several Islamic principles involved in dissecting the issue. Concerns regarding some vaccines not being halal originate from the use of porcine-based-enzymes in their production. The Islamic Fatwa Committee has allowed the usage of these vaccines.[30]

HUMAN FOETUSES ABORTED TO PRODUCE VACCINES

Vaccine research and production requires culturing of the virus in specific human cells. Rumours were spread that human foetuses are aborted to produce vaccines. However, this is not true. The process now uses laboratory-produced human cell-line culture, but historically, these cells were harvested from medically terminated human foetuses.[30]

RELIGION: AN INSTRUMENT TO WHIP UP VACCINE HESITANCY

Opposition to vaccines on religious grounds, though largely unfounded, started with the discovery of vaccines and continues unabated. When smallpox vaccination commenced, some of its opponents argued that if God had decreed someone's death from smallpox, it would be a sin to thwart God's will.

Another popular religious prejudice against vaccination is the use for cell culture media of some viral vaccines derived from tissues taken from therapeutic abortions performed on human foetuses in the 1960s. Moreover, Islamic clerics have been opposing vaccines, alleging that they are made with pork gelatine. Rumours that the polio vaccine contains pig's blood were also common.[25]

Another rumour spread about vaccines is that they weaken the immune system. Rumours that they do not prevent diseases were also prevalent.

EPIDEMIC OF DISTRUST

Vaccines are developed by a complicated process and require trust in the government, healthcare providers and the scientific community. Breach of trust in even one of these makes it difficult to convince people to be vaccinated.

Scholars have reported that vaccine hesitancy is a manifestation of growing public distrust in public health authorities and organized medicine.[3,24] A reduced trust in allopathy and a growing interest in natural products and alternative medicine is also resulting in vaccine hesitancy.[32]

It is very important to identify and understand the drivers of distrust to design interventions and strategies to build trust in vaccines.[24]

VICTIMS OF THEIR OWN SUCCESS

Due to serious and sometimes fatal consequences of diseases, most vaccines have been welcomed with great enthusiasm. Gradually, due to the success of immunization, morbidity and mortality associated with the diseases has faded from public memory. Consequently, parents and health professionals lack first-hand knowledge of the risks of contracting such diseases. A sense of complacency prevails, which has been termed by the WHO as one of the most influential determinants of vaccine hesitancy.[11,33]

Thus, when vaccines are successful, they become their own worst enemy.[3] Consequently, some well-controlled vaccine-preventable diseases have staged a comeback.[3]

ROLE OF POLITICAL ACTORS AND CELEBRITIES

Politicians and celebrities play a critical role in allaying and fuelling vaccine hesitancy. A famous example is of the British Prime Minister Tony Blair. When asked in 2002 whether he had given the MMR vaccine to his youngest son, he did not give a clear answer. This fuelled speculation about the vaccine's safety and intensified the ongoing MMR-autism debate.[3]

Anti-vaxxers also found support in US President Donald Trump. He not only openly supported a concept of the MMR-Autism linkage but also invited Andrew Wakefield to attend his inaugural balls. His tweet in 2014, 'A healthy young child goes to the doctor, gets pumped with massive shot of many vaccines, doesn't feel good and changes—AUTISM' was a shot in the arms of anti-vaxxers.[34]

The list also features Heather Whitestone, a young deaf woman, who was crowned Miss America in 1994. In a pre-pageant interview, she told media that she had lost her hearing as a toddler after 'strong medication' was given to her to treat a high fever resulting from the DPT vaccine. The story was morphed by anti-vaxxers who published reports ascribing Ms. Whitestone's disability to a near-fatal reaction to DTP vaccination.[3]

PREFERRING THE PANDEMIC TO VACCINES

In 2020, the world was devastated by the COVID-19 pandemic. When the inoculations started, some people did not see the vaccine as a silver bullet. The development of COVID-19 vaccines at an unprecedented speed and consequent worries about their safety and efficacy were the main reasons for vaccine hestancy.[33,35] Lack of accessibility and transparency of data and information about vaccine safety and efficacy led to vaccine hesitancy.[37,38] Initial surveys in Canada, the United Kingdom and the USA found that fewer than 60 per cent of the participants were ready to take the COVID vaccine.[38,39]

The anxieties, doubts and uncertainties were amplified by misinformation campaigns. These included older narratives that vaccines are used to sterilize people and have major side effects; the harmless nature of the virus; the existence of natural immunity; not being enough at risk from COVID-19, and utmost belief in God. Religious misconceptions such as vaccines containing tissues from aborted foetuses or traces of pork or cow meat had also resurfaced.[40,41]

New rumours were manufactured too such as vaccines being used to insert microchips in people's bodies, permanently altering their genes, damaging their DNA or even turning them into monkeys.[40,41,42]

INDIA FIGHTS COVID-19 VACCINE HESITANCY

People's COVID-19 vaccine hesitancy was also a major challenge for India. The rushed launch of vaccines and lack of safety- and efficacy-related data perpetuated vaccine hesitancy. Low confidence in the health service, lack of adequate information, and fever after vaccination also contributed to this hesitancy.

Health workers battled misconceptions, conspiracy theories and physical assault. Being infected by the virus after vaccination also drove people away. 'In some asymptomatic cases, vaccination was linked by people to to flare-up of the disease and even deaths', said Dr Dhawal, Public Health Specialist in Dadra and Nagar Haveli.

'The medical fraternity and the highly literate community had low confidence in COVID-19 vaccines due to their variable efficacy and unknown long-term effects on the body', said Akhil Arora, Principle Secretary, Health and Family Welfare, Rajasthan.

As per Dr Devansh, Deputy Commissioner, Changlang, Arunachal Pradesh, 'Pregnant women and lactating mothers shunned COVID-19 vaccination as they feared severe adverse health effects on their babies'. He also told me that many people with co-morbidities were frightened of severe adverse reactions from the vaccine.

The vaccination drive was also stonewalled on religious grounds. For example, in Malana, a village in the Himalayas in northern India, the village council told people that the local deity, Jagadamani Rishi, also known as Jamlu Devta, had not agreed to it.

Misconceptions tagged to religion were also breeding vaccine hesitancy. 'Vaccine hesitancy in a community in my district was due to people thinking that some of the ingredients in the vaccines were extracted from pork', said Dr Meenu Meena, District Immunization Officer of Delhi's Central district.

WORLD WIDE WEB ENCOURAGES VACCINE HESITANCY

The internet, also called by some a 'modern Pandora's box', has transformed ways of acquiring knowledge.[11] It has now become an important source of health-related information.

The internet has also brought together individuals and groups who are critical of vaccines. Early anti-vaxxer pamphlets have been replaced by websites, blogs, email lists and related media.[43] The internet has enabled a minority of users to generate a disproportionate amount of anti-vaccination content and disseminate rumours, myths and misinformation. According to Betsch et al., even a brief exposure to vaccine-critical websites increases the overall perception of vaccine risk.[44]

The internet has also led to the significant growth of online research publications in the lack of a check on their quality and accountability. Anti-vaxxers post articles with accentuated titles and quickly readable text with dramatic but false anecdotes.[11] Furthermore, anti-vaccine websites are optimized to appear high on the results for vaccine-related internet searches.[3]

SOCIAL MEDIA: A SHOT IN THE ARM FOR ANTI-VAXXERS

The advent of smartphones and access to technology has led to the emergence and global penetration of social media platforms such has Facebook, Google, LinkedIn, Twitter and YouTube. Ease of operation has made these a popular means to voice opinions, provide advice and share text, photographs and videos.

However, it has also created a huge potential for spread of misinformation and conspiracy theories transnationally.[45] 'Digital wildfires' are the new tools for disrupting immunization-related efforts.[26] Anti-vaccination activists use vivid narratives, powerful imagery and manipulated videos to propagate misinformation on social media.[46] Users, especially those with cognitive impairment, older people and those with low literacy (as well as digital literacy) are vulnerable to such emotional appeals.[47]

Non-human run accounts such as 'bots' and 'trolls' are also being used to pollute content and amplify the anti-vaccination movement.[44] The WHO has also issued a warning that the world is battling an 'infodemic' that spreads fake news, information and scientific claims.

Misinformation unleashed by social media has been posing a formidable challenge to COVID-19 vaccination managers and governments. As per Dr Muthamma, Health Secretary, Dadra and Nagar Haveli and Daman and Diu, 'misinformation through social media is one of the prominent forces driving vaccine hesitancy.

We had to launch a large myth-busting campaign through social media to counter it'. She also circulated videos of prominent personalities taking a shot along with their messages on social media to counter the onslaught of misinformation.

A similar problem was shared with me by Amit Satija, Health Secretary, Lakshadweep: 'News circulated in social media claiming the vaccines were ineffective and just an eye wash for the public turned out to be a mammoth problem'. Dr Partiban, Health Secretary, Arunachal Pradesh faced similar challenges.

VACCINE EQUITY: A MUST FOR HEALTH AND ETHICAL REASONS

It has been established that new health interventions including vaccines follow 'inverse equity'. They initially favour the more privileged. HICs use product development partnerships and advanced market commitments to bring new products from the bench to the bedside quickly.[49]

The inverse equity hypothesis for vaccines applies both within and between countries and is a daunting public health challenge. Vaccine inequity is critical because the protective shield of vaccines works the best when everyone is vaccinated.

It is vital to understand and address the challenges posed by vaccine inequity while rolling out new vaccines. Strategies that ignore equity risk undermine the effectiveness of vaccination as a tool to control VPDs and have health-related and economic repercussions. The longer a pandemic lasts, the higher are the chances of more virulent and transmissible mutants.

Apart from the availability of vaccines, vaccine equity is also challenged by vaccine hesitancy, lack of storage capacities and delivery mechanisms, vaccine wastage, lack of grants for research, soaring vaccine prices, and lack of equity in vaccine-related communication.[50]

ELUSIVE VACCINE EQUITY IN SWINE FLU OUTBREAK

Before COVID-19, outbreaks of H1N1 (swine flu) demonstrated that LICs and LMICs find themselves the last in line when vaccines are required to control infectious diseases.

Swine flu originated in mid-April 2009 and efforts were initiated to develop a vaccine. Even before H1N1 was declared a pandemic on 11 June 2009, many HICs had signed pre-production agreements with potential manufacturers to advance purchase of all doses of H1N1 vaccines.[51]

This severely curtailed the access to vaccines of LMICs and 284,000 people died before the pandemic began to wane. Only at that stage did HICs pledge to donate 10 per cent of their vaccine doses. This was, however, portrayed as a much-needed goodwill gesture![51]

CHASING COVID-19 VACCINE EQUITY GLOBALLY

SARS-CoV-2 struck in early 2020 and brought havoc globally. An affordable and efficacious vaccine was considered the most potent tool to quell the pandemic. Equitable access to vaccines was critical to decimate the demon quickly.

National governments were in a dilemma about whether they should secure adequate doses of vaccines to meet their own domestic needs or procure them through global and equitable vaccine access. Despite their knowing that vaccine equity was in the self-interest of all countries and that 'no one was safe until everyone was safe', countries preferred the first alternative.

Even before the first vaccine secured EUA, HICs with only 14 per cent of the global population had reserved over half of pre-market purchase commitments of COVID-19 vaccines.[52] They had reserved more than one vaccine per person for their population.

To hedge their risks, these countries have invested in multiple vaccine candidates, leaving LICs and LMICs with no or inadequate vaccines to vaccinate even their high-risk populations.[53]

By 15 April 2021, 86 per cent of the 660 million vaccines had been administered to people in HICs and upper-middle-income countries (UMICs). The share of LICs was a mere 0.1 per cent. By 9 August 2020, people in LICs had only been vaccinated with 12.6 million of the 4.46 billion vaccines provided globally.[54]

Can international borders stop the spread of infectious diseases such as COVID-19? Even if HICs had inoculated their entire population, the contagion would have replicated rampantly in unvaccinated countries, with more potent and infectious mutations, which could escape both vaccines and natural immunity. Moreover, the recovery of national economies is dependent on resumption of stable global supply chains, opening up of global markets and reopening of international travel.[54,55]

Dr Tedros Adhanom Ghebreyesus, Director-General, WHO, expressed his serious concern about global vaccine inequity and called it 'a catastrophic moral failure whose price will be paid with the lives and livelihood of the poorest countries'.[53] The UN Secretary-General, Antonio Guterres, also sharply criticized the 'wildly uneven and unfair distribution' of COVID-19 vaccines. He said to the UN Security Council: 'Vaccine equity is the biggest moral test before the global community'.[54]

Several mechanisms were put in place to ensure cooperation, mobilize funds and converge efforts towards equitable availability of COVID-19 vaccines globally.

ACCESS TO COVID-19 TOOLS ACCELERATOR (ACT-A)

ACT-A was a collaborative platform led by the WHO, which was set up in April 2020 to speed up development and equitable distribution of healthcare products, including vaccines, to hasten the end of the COVID-19 pandemic. Its mandate was to coordinate financing and strategy, and the work of multiple global health partners. It had four pillars: diagnostics, therapeutics, vaccines and health systems.

However, it had inherent flaws. Its funding was based on an international aid model, which was dependent on the benevolence of donors.

COVID-19 TECHNOLOGY ACCESS POOL (C-TAP)

C-TAP was based on an open-science ideal and the values of social solidarity, international co-operation and shared responsibility. It was launched by the WHO in partnership with the Government of Costa Rica in May 2020. It was a voluntary multilateral pooling platform for sharing IPR, data, cell lines related to COVID-19 vaccines, diagnostics and medicines. It focused on scaling up of manufacturing capacity of vaccines and other crisis-relevant technologies in LMICs.[56]

However, only 41 countries supported C-TAP publicly. Support from the HICs was limited. Not a single company utilized the transfer process and the pool remained empty.[56] The WHO faced criticism for not promoting C-TAP, the lack of leadership in C-TAP and non-clarity on funds committed.[56]

COVAX: COVID-19 VACCINES GLOBAL ACCESS INITIATIVE

COVAX, the vaccine pillar of ACT-A, was born in April 2020 to cater to concerns that when COVID-19 vaccine production started, they would be garnered by rich countries. According to the Director General of the WHO, 'The COVAX facility is intended to ensure that the race for vaccines is collaboration, not a contest.'

COVAX, spearheaded by the WHO, with support from many other international organizations, was envisaged as a risk-sharing, resource-pooling and push financing mechanism. It aimed to mobilize funds to accelerate research and development of vaccines, stimulate investment in vaccine manufacturing, and facilitate equitable access to COVID-19 vaccines.

Under COVAX, countries were classified as 'self-funded' or 'funded'. Self-funded countries, which were mainly HICs, were asked to make upfront payment and a commitment to purchase allocated vaccines through the COVAX facility. Their contribution was partly used to cover investment in vaccines for poor countries. There was no restriction on the self-funded countries on their negotiations to purchase vaccines from different manufacturers.[56]

There were advantages for HICs in joining COVAX because this included hedging their vaccine procurement, and diversifying their vaccine portfolios at a time when there was no guarantee of the success of any vaccine candidate. Moreover, because of high-volume orders, the prices of vaccines were likely to come down.

While rich countries could access vaccines for 10 per cent to 50 per cent of their population, depending on the amount they paid, the access of poor countries to vaccines was limited to 20 per cent of their population, with allotted vaccinations in proportion to their population. After the 20 per cent threshold was reached, allocation depended on the public health vulnerabilities of a country.

By late September 2020, 92 LICs and LMICs and 54 HICs had joined COVAX. However, COVAX failed to muster universal support. Some of the most powerful countries favoured a nationalistic approach and bilateral purchase agreements.[57] COVAX was plagued by supply and funding shortfalls as well.

Many self-financing countries, although they made donations to COVAX, did not commit themselves to procuring vaccines through it. COVAX was also criticized for its lack of mechanisms for the enablement of technology transfer and IP sharing to enable

LMICs to produce their own vaccines. Moreover, its goal to reach 20 per cent of the population by the end of 2021 was modest.

However, despite major omissions and commissions, COVAX has set a historic precedent in public health and is the only mechanism that provides vaccine access to LICs. By the end of 2021, it had supplied over a billion doses of COVID-19 vaccines to 144 countries and territories. As per GAVI, nearly 90 per cent of these vaccines have gone to 92 LMICs.[58]

INTELLECTUAL PROPERTY RIGHT (IPR) WAIVER

Once the COVID-19 vaccine became a reality, humanity faced another formidable challenge. How the world would get at least 12 billion vaccine doses that were needed to achieve herd immunity? It was much beyond the capacity of patent-owning drug companies. IP rights were the main obstruction to expanding production.

Article IX of the Agreement, which had established the WTO, states that 'in exceptional circumstances, the Ministerial Conference may decide to waive an obligation imposed on a Member by this Agreement or any of the Multilateral Trade Agreements'. So India and South Africa moved a proposal to the WTO to suspend initially for three years certain IP obligations of pharma companies for health products and technologies, including vaccines, required for 'prevention, containment or treatment of COVID-19'.

The waiver aimed to facilitate production of vaccines in LMICs.[56] It was expected that the waiver would also push companies with patents to ramp up their supplies.

In April 2021, a group of 170 former heads of states and governments, and Nobel Laureates put their weight behind the proposal. However, despite being backed by over 100 countries in the WTO, and a concerted global campaign initiated by civil society, the proposal was blocked repeatedly by select HICs.

The HICs' point of view was that the waiver was not a panacea because LMICs lacked the capacity to produce vaccines and that raw material was in short supply.[59] However, this argument is specious, since many LMICs including India have the ability to ramp up vaccine production rapidly.

On 5 May 2021, the USA announced its support, although for a narrower version of the waiver, for vaccines only. This shifted the political lines and prompted support from other world leaders too.[56]

A THIRD WAY: TECHNOLOGY TRANSFER HUBS

A 'third-way', apart from the proposed IP waiver and private licensing, to achieve global COVID-19 vaccine equity was suggested in February 2021 by Ngozi Okonjo-Iweala, Director-General of the WTO. His suggestion was related to facilitation of technology transfer within the ambit of multilateral rules.

However, the proposal was devoid of details. Prima facie it seemed similar to C-TAP. Naturally, it faced opposition from vaccine license-holders. Some activists suspected that the third way was only an endeavour to halt the momentum built by the IP waiver proposal.

NATIONAL VACCINE EQUITY

Equitable access to vaccines for people within a country is critical for combating VPDs. However, it does not mean equal access, irrespective of age, health status and exposure-related risk. Development of vaccine delivery infrastructure and systems is also critical for equitable vaccines.[55]

The risk of contracting the disease, and the severity of illness and death rates depend on multiple biological, social and economic factors.[55] These factors must be taken into account in prioritization of population sub-groups to receive vaccines.

A contentious issue is whether older adults and people with serious medical conditions or the essential workers should be prioritized? The former category has the greatest risk of severe health outcomes, including death. The latter, due to their large number of interpersonal contacts, are at the greatest risk of infection and transmission. Therefore, targeting them is a viable strategy to bring down the number of cases.[55] In the case of new vaccines that are shrouded in uncertainty about their effectiveness and delivery constraints, increased benefits may ensue by prioritizing the elderly.

During the COVID-19 pandemic, countries formulated prioritization strategies to achieve intra-nation vaccine equity. India followed the prioritization strategy recommended by the NEGVAC. The guidelines aimed to maximize the overall public good, taking into account both health and non-health outcomes.

VACCINE NATIONALISM: 'MY COUNTRY FIRST'

The efforts of countries to secure priority access to emerging vaccines are known as vaccine nationalism.[58] Resourceful governments usually deploy geo-economic strategies such as APAs or advance market commitments (AMCs) even before vaccines are licenced.[60] This approach disrupts the equitable global distribution of vaccines.

When the COVID-19 pandemic struck in early 2020, countries scrambled to stockpile vaccines for their citizens. HICs reserved millions of vaccines for their domestic use even before any vaccine had passed clinical trials.[61] Governments also banned export of vaccines and the critical raw materials needed to produce them.[58] Vaccine nationalism also bred fierce competition among the HICs.

Although vaccine nationalism garnered press headlines during the COVID-19 pandemic, it is not a novel concept. It was at play during earlier pandemics such as H1N1.

Vaccine nationalism undermines efforts to treat vaccines as a global public good and poses a threat to fair and equitable distribution of vaccines. It is considered a short-sighted, risky, morally indefensible and inefficient approach.[58,60] It impedes economic recovery, hampers international cooperation and causes geopolitical tension. Moreover, the competition to buy vaccines pushes up their price.

As rightly said by the Director-General of the WHO in the context of the COVID-19 pandemic, 'Vaccine nationalism only helps the virus.... In the COVID-19 vaccine race, we either win together or lose together'. United Nations Secretary General Antonio Guterres tweeted on 3 January 2021: 'Vaccine nationalism is not only unfair, it is self-defeating. No country will be safe until all countries are safe'.

VACCINE EAGERNESS: THE OTHER SIDE OF THE COIN

Vaccine eagerness poses an equally huge challenge. Initially, a new vaccine is generally met with eagerness. Therefore, it is critical to manage and mitigate the disappointment of people who fail to secure a vaccination.

Vaccine eagerness soars in a pandemic. People are keen not only to get a protective shield against the disease, but they are also desperate to get back to normal life. Therefore, campaign managers need to tackle vaccine eagerness. It is vital to generate awareness and provide correct, consistent and timely information to the community to drive home the logic behind the prioritization of certain age or occupation groups for vaccination.

In the case of COVID-19 vaccines, their limited supply in the initial phase and the disastrous health-related consequences of the disease led to vaccine eagerness. In India, instances of people gathering at vaccination centres and opting for fake medical certificates regarding co-morbidities to jump the queue were reported.

The Prime Minister Modi was quick to recognize the consequences of vaccine eagerness. That is why he not only took the vaccination, based on his turn, but also advised other political leaders to do so.

Amidst the waves of vaccine hesitancy and vaccine eagerness, and pro-vax and anti-vax movements, countries also used COVID-19 vaccinations as diplomatic arsenals. As soon as it rolled out its vaccination drive, India emerged as a star player in vaccine diplomacy. The next chapter, elaborates India's 'Vaccine Maitri' programme and the vaccine diplomacy efforts of other countries.

REFERENCES

1. Gopalakrishnan S, Sujitha P. Vaccine hesitancy in India—the challenges: A review. *International Journal of Community Medicine and Public Health.* 2020 November 7;7(11):4643.
2. World Health Organization. Ten threats to global health in 2019. Available from: https://www.who.int/newsroom/spotlight/ten-threats-to-global-health in 2019
3. Chatterjee A, editor. Vaccinophobia and vaccine controversies of the 21st century. New York, NY: Springer; 2013.
4. Lo NC, Hotez PJ. Public health and economic consequences of vaccine hesitancy for measles in the United States. *JAMA Pediatrics.* 2017 September 1;171(9):887–892.
5. Cherian V, Saini NK, Sharma AK, Philip J. Prevalence and predictors of vaccine hesitancy in an urbanized agglomeration of New Delhi, India. *Journal of Public Health.* 2022 March;44(1):70–76.
6. Dubé E, Gagnon D, Zhou Z, Deceuninck G. Parental vaccine hesitancy in Quebec (Canada). *PLoS Currents.* 2016 March 7;8.
7. Machingaidze S, Wiysonge CS. Understanding COVID-19 vaccine hesitancy. *Nature Medicine.* 2021 August;27(8):1338–9.
8. Sage Working Group. (2014). Strategic advisory group of experts on immunization. Available from: https://www.who.int/immunization/sage/meetings/2014/october/1_Report_WORKING_GROUP_vaccine_hesitancy_final.pdf
9. Dubé E, M Vivion, N E MacDonald. Vaccine hesitancy, vaccine refusal and the anti-vaccine movement: influence, impact and implications. Expert review of vaccines. 2 January 2015.14(1):99–117.
10. MacDonald NE. Vaccine hesitancy: Definition, scope and determinants. *Vaccine.* 2015 August 14;33(34):4161–4164.

11. Petrelli F, Contratti CM, Tanzi E, Grappasonni I. Vaccine hesitancy, a public health problem. *Ann Ig*. 2018 March 1;30(2):86–103.
12. Orient JM. Vaccine Controversies: the Case for Freedom and Informed Consent. *Journal of American Physicians and Surgeons*. 2019;24(3).
13. Spier RE. Perception of risk of vaccine adverse events: a historical perspective. Vaccine. 2001 October 15;20:S78–84.
14. Prabhu M. The long view: Ye olde anti-vaxxers [Internet]. GAVI.org. 2021 [cited 7 September 2021]. Available from: https://www.gavi.org/vaccineswork/long-view-ye-olde-anti-vaxxers
15. François G, Duclos P, Margolis H, Lavanchy D, Siegrist CA, Meheus A, et al. Vaccine safety controversies and the future of vaccination programs. *The Pediatric Infectious Disease Journal*. 2005 Nov 1;24(11):953–961.
16. Vaccination—medical history of British India. National Library of Scotland [Internet]. Digital.nls.uk. 2021 [cited 7 October 2021]. Available from: https://digital.nls.uk/indiapapers/vaccination.html
17. Explained. The history of vaccine opposition in India—the case of smallpox [Internet]. *The Indian Express*. 2021 [cited 7 October 2021]. Available from: https://indianexpress.com/article/explained/covid-vaccine-opposition-history-india-7201266/
18. History of Indian opinion. Articles on and by Gandhi [Internet]. Mkgandhi.org. 2021 [cited 7 October 2021]. Available from: https://www.mkgandhi.org/articles/history-of-indian-opinion.html
19. Brimnes N. Fallacy, sacrilege, betrayal and conspiracy: The cultural construction of opposition to immunisation in India. In *The politics of vaccination: A global history*. Manchester: Manchester University Press; 2017.
20. Basharat S. Vaccine hesitancy through the ages: A glimpse into the past and the plague in British India. Available from: https://www.reviewofreligions.org/27938/vaccine-hesitancy-through-the-ages-a-glimpse-into-the-past-and-the-plague-in-british-india/
21. Plotkin SA, editor. *History of vaccine development*. Berlin: Springer Science & Business Media; 2011.
22. Maguire W. Early immunisation as a preventive measure against tuberculosis. *The Journal of State Medicine* (1912–1937). 1929 July 1;37(7):421–427.
23. Fitzpatrick M. The cutter incident: How America's first polio vaccine led to a growing vaccine crisis. *Journal of the Royal Society of Medicine*. 2006 March;99(3):156.
24. Lasco G, Yu VG. Communicating COVID-19 vaccines: Lessons from the dengue vaccine controversy in the Philippines. *BMJ Global Health*. 2021 March;6(3):e005422.
25. Agrawal A, Kolhapure S, Di Pasquale A, Rai J, Mathur A. Vaccine Hesitancy as a challenge or vaccine confidence as an opportunity for childhood immunisation in India. *Infectious Diseases and Therapy*. 2020 Sep;9(3):421–432.

26. Yach D. Issues in ensuring COVID-19 vaccine compliance—Foundation for a smoke-free world [Internet]. Foundation for a Smoke-Free World. 2021 [cited 7 October 2021]. Available from: https://www.smokefreeworld.org/issues-in-ensuring-covid-19-vaccine-compliance/
27. Kumar D, Chandra R, Mathur M, Samdariya S, Kapoor N. Vaccine hesitancy: understanding better to address better. *Israel Journal of Health Policy Research*. 2016 Dec;5(1):1–8.
28. Wilson SL, Wiysonge C. Social media and vaccine hesitancy. *BMJ Global Health*. 2020 October 1;5(10):e004206.
29. Hannigan J. Vaccine controversies. NU Writing. 2014(5).
30. Ali A. Childhood vaccine controversies: the myths, the facts and the uncertainties. *Scientific Malaysian*. 2016 June 13;12.
31. DeStefano F, Bodenstab HM, Offit PA. Principal controversies in vaccine safety in the United States. *Clinical Infectious Diseases*. 2019 Aug 1;69(4):726–731.
32. Siddiqui M, Salmon DA, Omer SB. Epidemiology of vaccine hesitancy in the United States. *Human Vaccines & Immunotherapeutics*. 2013 December 24;9(12):2643–2648.
33. Kekatos M. Nearly 80% of Americans think that the speedy approval process of a coronavirus vaccine is driven by politics–not by proof that shots work [Internet]. The Harris Poll. 2020 [cited 20 January 2022]. Available from: https://theharrispoll.com/nearly-80-of-americans-think-that-the-speedy-approval-process-of-a-coronavirus-vaccine-is-driven-by-politics-not-by-proof-that-shots-work/
34. U.S. public now divided over whether to get COVID-19 vaccine [Internet]. Pew Research Center Science & Society. 2021 [cited 7 October 2021]. Available from: https://www.pewresearch.org/science/2020/09/17/u-s-public-now-divided-over-whether-to-get-covid-19-vaccine/
35. Petrelli F, Contratti CM, Tanzi E, Grappasonni I. Vaccine hesitancy, a public health problem. *Ann Ig*. 2018 March;30(2):86–103.
36. Silberner J. Calling Dr Trump. *British Medical Journal* [Online]. 2019 December 9; 367.
37. Mallapaty S, Ledford H. COVID-vaccine results are on the way—and scientists' concerns are growing. 2020 [cited 25 December 2020]. Available from: https://www.nature.com/articles/d41586-020-02706-6
38. Talev M. Axios-Ipsos poll: America turns against coronavirus vaccine [Internet]. Axios. 2021 [cited 7 October 2021]. Available from: https://www.axios.com/axios-ipsos-poll-coronavirus-index-vaccine-doubts-e9205f29-8c18-4980-b920-a25b81eebd84.html
39. Robertson E, Reeve KS, Niedzwiedz CL, Moore J, Blake M, Green M, Katikireddi SV, Benzeval MJ. Predictors of COVID-19 vaccine hesitancy in the UK household longitudinal study. *Brain, Behavior, and Immunity*. 2021 May 1;94:41–50. Available from: https://www.medrxiv.org/content/10.1101/2020.12.27.20248899v1

40. Abbas Q, Mangrio F, Kumar S. Myths, beliefs, and conspiracies about COVID-19 Vaccines in Sindh, Pakistan: An online cross-sectional survey. Authorea Preprints. 2021 Mar 8. Available from: https://doi.org/10.22541/au.161519250.03425961/v1
41. *India Today* Web Desk. Debunking myths related to Covid-19 vaccines. *India Today*. [cited 29 January 2021). Available from: https://www.indiatoday.in/information/story/debunking-myths-related-to-covid-19-vaccines-1763959-2021-01-29
42. Loomba A, de Figueiredo SJ, Piatek K, de Graaf H, Larson J. Measuring the impact of exposure to COVID-19 vaccine misinformation on vaccine intent in the UK and US. *Nature Human Behaviour*. Available from: https://doi.org/10.1038/s41562-021-01056-1
43. Aggarwal A. Faith or safety? Covid vaccines spark religious concerns over pork gelatin, cow blood. *India Today*. 2020 December 28. Available from: https://www.indiatoday.in/coronavirus-outbreak/vaccine-updates/story/religious-hurdle-for-covid-19-vaccines-religious-leaders-raise-concern-over-pork-gelatin-cow-blood-in-vaccines-1753992-2020-12-28
44. Betsch C, Renkewitz F, Betsch T, Ulshöfer C. The influence of vaccine-critical websites on perceiving vaccination risks. Journal of health psychology. 2010 Apr;15(3):446–455.
45. Nair AT, Nayar KR, Koya SF, Abraham M, Lordson J, Grace C, Sreekumar S, Chembon P, Swarnam K, Pillai AM, Pandey AK. Social media, vaccine hesitancy and trust deficit in immunization programs: a qualitative enquiry in Malappuram District of Kerala, India. *Health Research Policy and Systems*. 2021 August;19(2):1–8.
46. Burki T. Vaccine misinformation and social media. *The Lancet Digital Health*. 2019 October 1; 1(6):e258–259.
47. Puri N, Coomes EA, Haghbayan H, Gunaratne K. Social media and vaccine hesitancy: new updates for the era of COVID-19 and globalized infectious diseases. *Human Vaccines & Immunotherapeutics*. 2020 November 1;16(11):2586–2593.
48. Broniatowski DA, Jamison AM, Qi S, AlKulaib L, Chen T, Benton A, Quinn SC, et al. Weaponized health communication: Twitter bots and Russian trolls amplify the vaccine debate. *American Journal of Public Health*. 2018 October;108(10):1378–84.
49. Ahonkhai V, Martins SF, Portet A, Lumpkin M, Hartman D. Speeding access to vaccines and medicines in low-and middle-income countries: a case for change and a framework for optimized product market authorization. PLoS One. 2016 Nov 16;11(11):e0166515.
50. Mitchell S, Andersson N, Ansari NM, Omer K, Soberanis JL, Cockcroft A. Equity and vaccine uptake: a cross-sectional study of measles vaccination in Lasbela District, Pakistan. *BMC International Health and Human Rights*. 2009 Oct;9(1):1–0.

51. Rutschman AS. The COVID-19 vaccine race: Intellectual property, collaboration(s), nationalism and misinformation. Wash. *UJL and Pol'y*. 2021;64:167.
52. Harman S, Erfani P, Goronga T, Hickel J, Morse M, Richardson ET. Global vaccine equity demands reparative justice—not charity. *BMJ Global Health*. 2021 June 1;6(6):e006504.
53. van de Pas R, Widdowson MA, Ravinetto R, Ochoa TJ, Fofana TO, Van Damme W. COVID-19 vaccine equity: A health systems and policy perspective. Available from: https://doi.org/10.1080/14760584.2022.2004125
54. Diseases TL. COVID-19 vaccine equity and booster doses. *The Lancet Infectious Diseases*. 2021 Sep;21(9):1193.
55. World Health Organization. WHO SAGE values framework for the allocation and prioritization of COVID-19 vaccination, 14 September 2020. World Health Organization. 2020.
56. Geiger S, McMahon A. Too many cooks or too many recipes? An analysis of the institutional landscape and proliferation of proposals for global vaccine equity for COVID-19. 11 March 2021.
57. COVAX vaccine roll-out [Internet]. GAVI.org. 2022 [cited 18 January 2022]. Available from: https://www.gavi.org/covax-vaccine-roll-out
58. Abbas MZ. Practical implications of vaccine nationalism: A short-sighted and risky approach in response to COVID-19. Research Paper. 2020.
59. Okereke M. Towards vaccine equity: Should big pharma waive intellectual property rights for COVID-19 vaccines? Public Health in Practice (Oxford, England). 2021 Nov;2:100165.
60. Rutschman AS. Is There a cure for vaccine nationalism? *Current History*. 2021 January;120(822):9–14.
61. Nigam S. Ensuring vaccine equity, erasing vaccine nationalism: Upholding the human rights and justice framework. 15 April 2021.

Chapter 8

India's Vaccine Diplomacy

The COVID-19 pandemic came with a new diplomatic currency: the COVID-19 vaccine. But is healthcare a novel diplomatic battlefield?

HEALTH DIPLOMACY

In recent decades, health has been ascendant in the foreign policy agendas of most developed and developing countries due to formidable challenges such as HIV/AIDS, other epidemics and pandemics, and the threat of bioterrorism.[1,2] Countries are increasingly using health diplomacy to extend their soft power, strengthen their diplomatic ties, cultivate deeper relationships with their citizens, and improve their image both at home and abroad.[3,4,5]

However, health is not new in the field of diplomacy. Cholera epidemics, which battered Europe in the 19th century, propelled disease control to the centre stage of diplomatic discussion. In 1851, France organized the first International Sanitary Conference to prevent the spread of cholera. Plague and yellow fever were added to the agenda in subsequent events.[6]

The increasing global threat of infectious diseases has led to the creation of conferences, treaties, processes and rules for global health governance and the creation of international health organizations to facilitate cooperation.[7] Countries realized that diseases were threats to economic development and national security and started using health diplomacy to advance their diplomatic goals.[8] The Oslo Declaration of foreign ministers in 2007 called upon governments to adopt a diplomatic approach that addresses public health concerns.[9]

Diplomatic discussions about epidemics intensified when SARS, the first global epidemic of the 21st century, struck in 2003. International health regulations were framed to address the slow response to the outbreak.[10] The swine flu epidemic, which infected more than 100 million people in 150 countries and killed 75,000 people from 2009 to 2018, saw more successful regional and bilateral initiatives.[11]

In the case of Ebola, which emerged in Guinea in early 2014, the United Nations took the lead, coordinated international efforts and set up the United Nations Mission for Ebola Emergency Response (UNMEER). A strong bilateral diplomatic effort was also made to contain the disease.[10]

COVID-19 saw the shifting of health diplomacy's centre of gravity away from rich countries and global institutions. This time, the aid flowed from the developing countries to the developed ones.

INDIA: A RISING STAR IN HEALTH DIPLOMACY

India's health diplomacy is powered by its strong pharmaceutical industry, which churns out 20 per cent of generic medicine and 62 per cent of vaccines produced globally; 67 per cent of the medicines manufactured in India are exported.[12] India's international reputation and goodwill soared when it supplied affordable anti-retroviral medicines to developing countries to fight the AIDS pandemic.[13]

Health diplomacy is an integral part of India's foreign policy. It stands on grants, soft loans, lines of credit with subsidized interest rates from the EXIM Bank, technical cooperation and contributions to international organizations. India's foreign assistance in the health sector is continuously on the rise.

India strongly believes in south-south cooperation. For geo-economic, geo-political and geostrategic reasons, Africa, the 'continent of the future', figures prominently in its health diplomacy agenda. India's diplomatic efforts include the supply of lifesaving drugs and pharmaceuticals, the transfer of technologies in healthcare, imparting education and training, and providing support to improve healthcare systems in African countries.[14]

INDIA: THE SAVIOUR OF THE WORLD IN COVID-19 PANDEMIC

The COVID-19 pandemic provided an opportunity for India to leverage its strengths in its pharmaceutical sector to enhance its reputation as a credible, neutral and trusted development partner.[15] To tackle the extraordinary challenge posed by the pandemic, Prime Minister Modi gave the age-old mantra, *Vasudeva Kutumbukam*—the world is one family.[16]

During the COVID-19 pandemic, India swiftly augmented its production of medical supplies such as hydroxychloroquine, remdesivir, paracetamol, diagnostic kits, ventilators, masks and PPE kits, and made them available to more than 150 countries.[17] It also sent rapid action teams and food grains to the developing countries.[18] As a part of the 'Mission Sagar' initiative, the Indian Naval ship, *INS Kesari*, with medical teams onboard, was pressed into service to deliver aid to countries in the Indian Ocean and help them with their COVID-19 management.

Unlike some countries that imposed export bans on essential medicine and equipment, India shared whatever it could with less well-off countries.[19] Its large-hearted approach and speedy response earned it accolades from countries and international organizations.[20,21]

India also launched a capacity-building programme for healthcare workers in South Asian and African countries.[22] Training courses on prevention and management of COVID-19 were organized for frontline healthcare workers as well. The Aarogya Setu and CoWIN apps were provided pro-bono to help in monitoring and management of the outbreak.

A CARING AND CONCERNED NEIGHBOUR

During the COVID-19 pandemic, as a caring neighbour, India made special efforts to reach out to its neighbours. Aside from medical supplies and food grains, it sent rapid action teams of medical professionals to assist them as the first respondent.[17]

On 15 March 2020, Prime Minister Modi convened a virtual meeting with the South Asian Association for Regional Cooperation (SAARC) to discuss regional efforts to control the pandemic by sharing resources, expertise, best practices and capacities. He also announced the creation of a SAARC COVID-19 emergency fund and India's contribution of $10 million to it.[23]

India also initiated the SAARC COVID-19 Information Exchange Platform (COINEX) to facilitate discussions, online training, knowledge partnerships, sharing of expertise and joint research on epidemic diseases.[17] Under its ITEC programme, India provided e-training to medical professionals in South Asian countries.[22] Its Vande Bharat mission evacuated citizens of its South Asian neighbours who were stranded in other countries.[17] India also proposed a special visa scheme for nurses and doctors in South Asia and the Indian Ocean Island countries.

TOUGH COMPETITOR IN THE NEIGHBOURHOOD

India faces stiff competition in health diplomacy from China, which is increasingly using public health to fortify its diplomatic relations with the developing world. China is also bolstering its influence in South Asia through economic and health engagements.[24,25]

Since the 1960s, Africa has been another focus area of Chinese health diplomacy. It started sending 'angels in white' and 'barefoot doctors' to African countries. Over the years, the country deepened its engagement with African countries and provided support to them on infrastructure, training of health practitioners and infectious disease prevention efforts.[26] Apart from projecting itself as a 'responsible state', China is using health diplomacy to expand its political and economic footprint and access natural resources on the African continent.[27]

When COVID-19 emerged in Wuhan and started spreading to the world, China was at the receiving end of its mishandling of the outbreak. In an endeavour to transform its image into that of a magnanimous global leader and a saviour, China donated PPE, masks and testing kits to countries around the world.[28,29,30] Although this earned them their gratitude, Chinese efforts were blemished by faulty gear supplied and resentment over its demand for effusive, publicly expressed gratitude.[31]

China also linked its COVID-19 medical supplies to its ambitious Belt and Road Initiative (BRI), which encompasses a large collection of investment and development initiatives extending from East Asia to Europe, which were launched in 2013. The linking of medical supplies to BRI was referred to as the 'health silk road'.[32,33]

VACCINES: NEW FRONTIERS IN INTERNATIONAL RELATIONS?

'Vaccine diplomacy' was a hot discussion topic during the COVID-19 pandemic. It involved creating a conducive environment for scientific collaboration for vaccine development and subsequent diplomatic activities relating to procurement and distribution of vaccines.[6,34]

Like other forms of diplomacy, vaccine diplomacy is undertaken to serve national interests and smoothen foreign relations. Many times, gift of vaccines come with geopolitical or economic strings attached. But such strings are kept under wraps. Vaccine diplomacy has been used by countries to burnish their soft power, display their technological prowess, please their domestic audiences and give their companies a firm foothold in new markets.

Vaccine diplomacy has been a known expression in the diplomatic dictionary since the discovery of the smallpox vaccine in 1798. Edward Jenner shipped his vaccine to many countries. He also provided these to France during the Anglo-French War.[35] He worked as an unofficial diplomat between Britain and France, and declared: 'The sciences are never at war'.

Britain used the smallpox vaccine to buy goodwill in its growing empire. As early as 1801, the USA used the smallpox vaccine to build diplomatic ties. Edward Gantt, the first White House physician, vaccinated Native American diplomats on their visit to Washington DC [36,37]

France became a pioneer in vaccine diplomacy after Louis Pasteur developed the rabies vaccine. The French Government built laboratories to produce and administer the vaccine on a mass scale throughout its colonies.[36] Vaccine diplomacy was even used during wars to mediate cessation of hostilities. Ceasefires were negotiated for vaccination campaigns.[37,38,39,40] Health assistance has been used in tandem with military intervention to win the hearts and minds of people.[41]

In today's world, countries are using their vaccine capacities to expand their spheres of political influence. Vaccine diplomacy has been at play during disease outbreaks, epidemics and pandemics.[42] Diplomatic interventions helped to overcome the call to boycott polio vaccination in Nigeria in 2003.[43] During the COVID-19 pandemic, apart from bilateral vaccine diplomacy, multilateral diplomacy was also evident throughout the COVAX facility.

BREACHING THE 'IRON CURTAIN'

In the 1950s, despite heightened tensions and the threat of nuclear war, the USA and the Soviet Union worked together to combat two menaces of that era: polio and smallpox.[44] For production and testing of the OPV, American virologist Dr Albert Sabin and Soviet virologist Dr Mikhail Chumakov worked together on two sides of the Iron Curtain.

A live OPV developed by Sabin had the potential to immunize millions of people much faster and at a lower cost than Jonas Salk's 'killed' vaccine. It was not feasible to test this vaccine on American children who had been vaccinated with Salk's vaccine. Sabin sent his virus strains to Chumakov who successfully tested it in 1959 on 10 million children across the Soviet Union.[37,45]

Thereafter, the two superpowers embarked on vaccine diplomacy and distributed the OPV around the world. It averted millions of deaths and disabilities and ultimately eliminated polio, except from Afghanistan and Pakistan.[36] The two superpowers also collaborated on eradicating smallpox. In the 1960s, Soviet scientists developed a freeze-dried smallpox vaccine and enabled its delivery to remote tropical areas.[46] The USA extended financial support for production and distribution of millions of doses of the vaccine globally. Their collaboration continued with a focus on tuberculosis and the prevention of HIV/AIDs and other sexually transmitted diseases.[47,48]

VACCINE: A SOFT POWER TOOL

In context of international relations, soft power is the ability of a country to attract and co-opt rather than coerce another country into shaping its preferences.[49] Inequity in access to vaccines has turned these into an instrument of soft power.[37] Countries are using vaccines as bargaining chips to further their national interests in the economic, political or security realms.

The COVID-19 pandemic made the vaccine against SARS-CoV-2 the most-in-demand commodity globally. National governments extensively used COVID-19 vaccines bilaterally to strengthen ties, better their global image, thaw frosty relations, reward old friends, make new friends, highlight the benefits of their ideologies and gain access to markets.[50]

When COVID-19 vaccine supplies were not forthcoming, the Philippine President Rodrigo Duterte threatened to terminate the Armed Forces Visiting Agreement with the USA.[51] Israel was allegedly made to finance an undisclosed number of Sputnik V vaccines by Russia to Damascus as ransom for the release of an Israeli civilian held in Syria.[52] China's vaccine donations were linked to pledges to oppose international intervention in China's internal affairs or support its Belt and Road Initiative.[53]

LEADERSHIP VACUUM DRIVES 'VACCINE MAITRI'

The COVID-19 pandemic was different. Epidemics and pandemics in the past mostly affected the global south. Therefore, support flowed from rich countries. However, the COVID-19 pandemic affected rich countries as well and led to a fierce competition among them to procure vaccines. Consequently, poor countries were left scrambling to secure supplies.[54]

The absence of the USA and other rich countries from vaccine diplomacy created a leadership vacuum. Therefore, countries in desperate need of vaccines turned to India and China to fill the void.[55]

India had a huge advantage in terms of its credibility and capability of developing and manufacturing vaccines. This provided it a unique opportunity to fill the vacuum and bolster its international image.

In his address at the 75th session of the UN General Assembly on 26 September 2020, Prime Minister Modi committed himself to using India's vaccine production capability to help humanity. 'As the largest vaccine-producing country in the world, I want to give one more assurance to the global community today. India's vaccine production and delivery capacity will be used to help all humanity in fighting this crisis', he told the world leaders.[56] Therefore, as soon as vaccines were approved by its regulator, India launched its ambitious diplomatic initiative 'Vaccine Maitri'.

VACCINE MAITRI

Vaccine Maitri, which means vaccine friendship, was kick-started on 21 January 2021, barely four days after commencement of India's domestic inoculation drive. Taking inspiration from the Sanskrit verse *Sarve Santu Niramaya* (may all be free from disease), millions of Indian-made COVID-19 vaccines were dispatched to over 100 countries.

Apart from its immediate neighbours, India's initial beneficiaries included its key Indian Ocean partners. Thereafter, India reached out to other developing countries. Commercial supply agreements were inked with many countries. India also made a huge contribution to COVAX.[57] Made in India vaccines were not only cheaper but were also more suitable for developing countries with weak infrastructure and cold chain facilities.

Rich countries, including Canada and the United Kingdom, also entered the queue for Indian vaccines. Canadian Prime Minister Justin Trudeau has made a request to Prime Minister Modi more than once to expedite supplies to Canada.[58]

It was a time of plummeting Chinese soft power due to 'strings attached' policy and the credibility-related crisis plaguing it. India leveraged its pharmaceutical power and quickly expanded Vaccine Maitri. By the end of 2021, it had supplied 117.31 million vaccines to 96 countries. This included 14.77 million bilateral free vaccines, 33.21 million vaccines sold to COVAX and 69.34 million vaccines supplied on bilateral commercial basis.[59,60,61] India took special care of the UN peacekeepers, presenting them with 200,000 COVID-19 vaccines.

NEIGHBOURHOOD FIRST

Vaccine Maitri was kicked off under India's policy of 'Neighbourhood First'. In the first round, India sent 0.55 million vaccines to Bhutan on 20 January 2021; 2 million vaccines to Bangladesh; 1.1 million vaccines to Nepal; 100,000 vaccines to the Maldives; 1.5 million vaccines to Myanmar, and 500,000 vaccines to Sri Lanka.[61,62]

By April 2021, India had sent 20 million vaccines to its neighbours, either free of cost or at their actual production cost. Apart from supplying vaccines, India also trained these countries' medical personnel and helped the countries strengthen their cold chain and storage capacities.[59] More than 2,400 people from 14 countries were trained. Their clinical trial capabilities were also strengthened under India's PACT initiative.[17]

The cost, speed of delivery and effectiveness of Indian vaccines threatened China, which had also offered vaccines to India's neighbours. However, these offers were declined by many countries due to the strings attached, lack of transparency and quality-related concerns.[59]

Vaccine Maitri bolstered India's credibility as a solution provider and a country that reacts promptly in times of crisis.[63] It also helped to create a positive impression of India among the people of its neighbouring countries. Vaccine Maitri provided an opportunity for India to counter the expanding political and economic influence of China in its neighbourhood.

Vaccine Maitri led to a thaw in India's strained relations with some of its neighbours. For example, it dissipated tension in Indo-Nepal relations that was generated over the political map of the Kalapani region. In the case of Bangladesh, aside from India's close ties with the country, Vaccine-Maitri won back the goodwill of people reportedly adversely affected by certain Indian policies.[63,64] In addition to its immediate neighbours, Vaccine Maitri also provided opportunities for India to build a strong diplomatic bond with Africa.

VACCINE MAITRI ON MULTILATERAL PLATFORMS

To control the devastating COVID-19 pandemic through vaccines, India extended help to a large number of low-income countries through multilateral platforms. It provided over 33 million vaccines to COVAX. India also vigorously pursued the vaccine patent waiver proposal at the WTO to enable production of COVID-19 vaccines at a fast pace in developing countries.

India has built a reputation of being a reliable manufacturer of high quality vaccines, a selfless contributor to global health and a vital node in global health supply chains. Therefore, when the QUAD, comprising of the USA, India, Japan and Australia, decided on 12 March 2021 to jointly develop, finance, distribute and manufacture vaccines, India was assigned the responsibility of producing one billion vaccines.[65,66]

After the first meeting of QUAD, Biological E. has entered an agreement with the US DFC to produce 1 billion doses of the Johnson & Johnson vaccine for export to the Indo-Pacific region by the end of 2022 under the QUAD framework. The initiative will be part funded by the US DFC. Another initiative under consideration under the QUAD framework is support of the Japan Bank for International Cooperation (JBIC) to upgrade the facilities of Gennova Biopharmaceuticals. This would enable India to expand its Vaccine Maitri scheme and strengthen its global standing.[67]

SANJEEVANIBOOTI GETS INTERNATIONAL ACCLAIM

Gratitude poured in for India's Vaccine Maitri. World leaders spoke warmly and appreciatively of the country's initiative to supply COVID-19 vaccines.

Brazil's President, Bolsonaro, sent his gratitude with an image from the Ramayana epic, depicting Lord Hanuman carrying an entire mountain of COVID-19 vaccine. He tweeted, 'Brazil feels honoured to have a great partner to overcome a global obstacle by joining our efforts'.[68]

Canada's President Trudeau declared that victory over COVID-19 would be 'because of India's tremendous pharmaceutical capacity and Prime Minister Modi's leadership in sharing this capacity with the world'. Antigua and Barbuda's Prime Minister, Gaston Alfonso Browne, called the delivery of Indian COVID-19 vaccines to the Caribbean countries 'an act of benevolence, kindness and empathy'. Praise also came from the USA: 'India is a true friend, using its pharma to help the global community'.

The WHO chief thanked Prime Minister Modi: 'Your commitment to #COVAX and sharing #COVID19 vaccines is helping more than 60 countries start vaccinating their health workers and other priority groups'. The United Nations chief, Antonio Guterres, appreciated India for bringing the 'much-needed supply' of the COVID-19 vaccines and for being a global leader in its response to the pandemic.

Microsoft founder Bill Gates also congratulated India. He tweeted: 'It's great to see India's leadership in scientific innovation and its vaccine manufacturing capability. India's role in vaccine production will be crucial to the whole world in combating the pandemic'.[69]

India's neighbours were full of praise for it. From Thimpu, Prime Minister Lotay Tshering expressed his gratitude: 'It is the display of altruism at its best. It's of unimaginable value when precious commodities are shared, even before meeting one's own needs'.[17]

Nepal's Prime Minister tweeted: 'I thank Prime Minister Shri @ narendramodi ji as well as the Government and people of India for their generous grant of one million COVID vaccines'. The Maldives' Foreign Minister Abdulla Shahid praised India's role as the first country that had responded to the country's call for help.

He said: 'As always, India stands strong and steadfast by our side in any crisis'.

The 79-member African, Caribbean and Pacific (ACP) group and the Caribbean Community (CARICOM) also praised Vaccine Maitri: 'This act of selflessness is a testament to the solidarity of the government and people of India with CARICOM'.

DID VACCINE MAITRI FORTIFY INDIA'S INTERNATIONAL IMAGE?

When India launched Vaccine Maitri, countries were scrambling for vaccines. Expressions such as *'vaccine race'*, *'vaccine apartheid'*, and *'vaccine nationalism'* had entered the global lexicon, but global cooperation in sharing vaccines was minimal. This situation presented India with the ideal opportunity to use its vaccine-manufacturing capacity to serve humanity and strengthen its international image.[70]

Vaccine Maitri catapulted India to the centre stage of global recovery from the COVID-19 pandemic. The initiative also created space for India in the hearts of people of more than 100 countries.[71,72] The quality of its vaccines added to India's credibility as a reliable vaccine producer.[73]

Coupled with health diplomacy, Vaccine-Maitri resulted in the Western countries seeing India as a counterbalancing force to the growing influence of China.[50,74] Vaccine Maitri also mended and deepened India's ties with its neighbours and strengthened its relations with the Indian Ocean and African countries.[59,75]

The world appreciated the rapidity and selflessness with which India rolled out millions of doses of COVID-19 vaccine, despite the massive requirements of its own vaccination drive.[76] As its External Affairs Minister Dr Jaishankar put it: 'Stressed and vulnerable nations of the world can see that there is at least one major nation that truly believes in making vaccines accessible and affordable to others in dire need'.[77]

Its massive diplomatic mission definitely projected India as a responsible global power and enhanced its global support and goodwill. For a long time to come, grateful governments will remember India's contribution to saving the world that was reeling from the onslaught of the deadly pathogen.[78]

The immense goodwill that Vaccine Maitri has earned will pay rich dividends in the future.[78] Increased trust and a feeling of gratitude will definitely help India realize its aspiration to secure permanent membership of the UN Security Council, whenever it is reformatted.

GENEROSITY AFFECTS INDIA

In April 2021, India was engulfed by the second wave of COVID-19. By then, it had inoculated less than 10 per cent of its people. There was a sudden spurt in the demand for vaccines, since the country had decided to roll out its COVID-19 vaccination programme universally. Consequently, Vaccine Maitri saw a temporary break.

India had exported more doses than it had used domestically. The Opposition accused the Government of being overzealous in its exports at the expense of its own people. As the country ran out of vaccines, people started asking: 'Did the Government miscalculate domestic requirements? Did India punch above its weight?'

Some countries also criticized India for reneging on its promises. And India temporarily lost a vital platform to gain traction and influence in South Asia and the developing world.[79] This gave China an opportunity to act on deepening its influence.[79]

However, export of vaccines is not a zero-sum game. Vaccines are perishable and need to be used before their expiry date. Therefore, when the domestic demand for vaccines was low, it was justified for the government to export vaccines to enhance India's international goodwill and global standing.[80]

THE DRAGON'S VACCINE DIPLOMACY

China's vaccine diplomacy was a continuation of its health-related diplomacy to address global mistrust and criticism over the origin and handling of SARS-CoV-2. It was also meant to be a financial booster for Chinese biotechnology companies.

With the USA busy buying a large number of vaccines for Americans, the power vacuum was a great geopolitical opportunity. China sounded the 'vaccine diplomacy' bugle with President Xi Jinping's announcement at the World Health Assembly's meeting in May 2020 that China considered its vaccines a 'global public good'.

By July 2020, clinical trials of Chinese vaccines had started in many developing countries. By November 2020, Chinese companies had struck deals to supply vaccines to some countries. In December 2021, Egypt became the first country to receive Chinese vaccines.[81]

Soon Chinese vaccines were all around the world, bolstering China's political allies. Surveys reported a dramatic increase in trust in China in countries obtaining Chinese vaccines. China was also ahead in transfer of technology and started manufacturing vaccines in 15 countries. This was welcomed because it gave a boost to the countries' pharmaceutical industries and created jobs in them.[82]

Although China distributed free vaccines to some countries, its commercial contracts were hundreds of times more than its donations. To help countries afford its vaccines, China extended them loans to buy these. Thus, it could extract favours from the recipients without the economic cost of donating vaccines. Moreover, the vaccines came with the strings of diplomatic and economic favours attached. China also sought to tie vaccine supplies to the advancement of its major BRI projects.

Chinese vaccine diplomacy was overwhelmingly bilateral and exceeded its committed contribution to COVAX, which it joined in October 2020 after its initial reluctance. Its decision was driven by economic considerations. Apart from this signalling China's support of multilateral institutions such as the WHO, its decision was an incentive for the WHO to approve Chinese vaccines.[83]

Moreover, China's vaccine diplomacy was aimed at softening the ill-will generated before the COVID-19 pandemic by geopolitical disputes such as its territorial claims in the South China Sea. China's efforts to dominate the World Bank and the IMF had also generated friction.[50]

However, the efficacy of Chinese vaccines was a major concern.[84] The WHO's studies revealed that China's Sinovac vaccine only prevented symptomatic disease in 51 per cent of those vaccinated.[85] The recipients of Chinese vaccines in various countries contracted COVID-19 even after receiving two shots.[86,87,88]

However, with wealthier countries opting for supplies of safer and more effective vaccines, China could easily push its less proven but affordable vaccines in LICs and LMICs, despite doubts about their effectiveness, and make these countries obligated to Beijing.

VACCINE MAITRI PAUSE: ADVANTAGE DRAGON

India had to temporarily suspend Vaccine Maitri due to a sudden peak in the domestic demand for vaccines due to the devastating second wave of COVID-19 in April and May 2021. This pause provided Beijing the opportunity to increase its influence in South Asian, Indo-Pacific and other developing countries. This also gave it the opportunity to pursue its BRI initiative.[63,89]

Suspension of Vaccine Maitri had consequences for countries expecting delivery of Indian vaccines. Although the spiralling health crisis made them extremely sympathetic to India, their search for alternative sources of vaccines led them to China.[51,90,91] This had potential strategic connotations for the region.[63]

Capitalizing on the urgency, China gifted 500,000 doses to Bangladesh on 12 May, 2021. However, this came with a warning the country was not to join the QUAD alliance.[63] The coercive overtone invited a strong response from Dhaka.[92] Other countries also benefited from Chinese vaccines.

To play a critical role in the COVID-19 end game and counter China's growing influence, especially in South Asia, it became imperative for India to resume Vaccine Maitri. The right time came in October 2021 when the COVID-19 peak was over and a large proportion of the Indian population had received at least one shot.[25] Vaccine Maitri-2.0 was kick-started again with supply of COVID-19 vaccines to Nepal, Bangladesh, Myanmar and Iran, although without much fanfare.[93]

MAHARAJA AND DRAGON: TWO NATIONS, TWO STYLES

During the COVID-19 crisis, both India and China were on a mission to win hearts, minds and influence, especially in the developing world. Aside from their regional rivalry, tensions between them had intensified during the COVID-19 pandemic following clashes along the Himalayan frontier.[94]

However, India and China differed in their strategies, ambition and operations. While India drew strength from its great manufacturing potential and lack of geo-political baggage, China had won the loyalty of countries with which it had close relations, built on economic cooperation and infrastructure projects.

China had explicitly demanded diplomatic, geopolitical and economic quid pro quos for its vaccines. It had reportedly put pressure on Paraguay to cut ties with Taiwan in exchange for vaccines and demanded that Brazil should reverse its plans to exclude Huawei from the upcoming 5G auctions.[83] Support for its Belt and Road Initiative and sharing the cost of vaccine trials with some of these countries were its other conditions.[95] India on the other hand did not expect anything material in return for its vaccines and even deployed special Air India flights to deliver the vaccines.

China distributed its vaccines globally by starting their production in collaboration with many countries including Brazil, Indonesia, Serbia and the United Arab Emirates. India's production largely remained domestic.[96]

India successfully overshadowed the dragon in its speed of delivery and the effectiveness of its vaccines. There were numerous examples of India's swiftness.[97] The efficacy of Chinese vaccines was found to be much lower than all other vaccines that were in use in the world. On the other hand, confidence in Indian vaccines made hem welcome even in rich countries, in contrast to Chinese products, which were largely confined to LICs and LMICs. Another difference was that while China was secretive in sharing data about its vaccines, India was open and transparent. It even organized trips for foreign ambassadors to see its pharmaceutical factories.

RUSSIAN VACCINE DIPLOMACY

Russia was another formidable competitor of India's Vaccine Maitri. On 11 August 2020, it became the first country with an approved COVID-19 vaccine. The vaccine was named Sputnik V, mirroring the name of the world's first artificial satellite, which the Soviet Union launched in 1957.

The vaccine initially received a lukewarm response because its Phase-2 clinical trials were only conducted on a limited number of people and the results of its Phase-3 clinical trials were awaited. It was only when its trial results were published in the *Lancet* that Sputnik V's prestige soared. With high efficacy and simple cold chain requirements, Sputnik V found favour with developing countries as well as in Europe.[98] This provided an opportunity for Russia to expand its influence in developing countries, enter into business deals with rich Western countries and promote itself as an Asian power.

Russia focused on bilateral deals with deliveries guided by its foreign policy and economic priorities. It focused on Latin America and opted for joint production of its vaccine in Brazil and Argentina.[51,99]

Russia also entered Africa, offering sale of vaccines along with a financial package to buy them. In Europe, Russia's offers of vaccine production or joint production were accompanied by messages about the European Union's failures.[88]

However, Russia's supplies were plagued with delays, causing an uproar in the recipient countries, tarnishing Russia's image.[100] Moreover, the price of Sputnik V was triple of the AstraZeneca vaccine.

FROM INWARD TO OUTWARD LOOKING: VACCINE DIPLOMACY OF THE USA

The USA has a rich history of vaccine diplomacy. However, it was slow to get out of the gate during the COVID-19 pandemic. This led to a narrative that an insular and battered US could not lead the world out of this crisis. The new US President, Biden, attempted to revitalize the image of US as an outward-looking, generous nation.[101]

The US had windows of opportunity to reclaim its leadership role in global health. These included a strong preference for its vaccines the world over, requirement for vaccines for years due to the long tail of the COVID-19 pandemic, efficacy issues with Chinese vaccines, supply issues with the Russian vaccine and the pause in India's Vaccine Maitri.[53,88]

The first change came with the US announcing its $4 billion support of COVAX and an appeal to its allies to donate their surplus vaccines. In June 2021, the US purchased 500 million vaccines for distribution by COVAX.[82] Initial supplies were destined for Latin America. The White House emphasized that no strings were attached to these donations. On 22 September 2021, President Biden pledged at the UN General Assembly that the USA would donate an additional 500 million doses through COVAX.[83,102]

The USA also pledged $370 million to support administration of its shots and $380 million to the Global Vaccine Alliance (GAVI) to handle distribution of its vaccines.[103] It also teamed up with India, Japan and Australia through the QUAD to provide billions of vaccines to developing countries. It is believed that it will outclass its competitors in the quality, scale and generosity of their donations in the medium and long term.

DIPLOMATIC FORAYS OF OTHER COUNTRIES

There were other players in the vaccine diplomacy space during the COVID-19 pandemic. Japan had pledged $1 billion to the COVAX facility and said that it would ship 23 million vaccines to various countries. It also supported the establishment of cold chains in developing countries.[104,105]

The United Arab Emirates played its vaccine diplomacy on the strength of its economic status, cutting-edge logistic sector and pivotal position between the East and the West.[106,107] It established a production centre for Sinopharm vaccines and rebranded it as Hayat-Vax (Hayat in Arabic meaning 'life') to create a perception that the initiative was an Emirati effort.[108] It has become one of the top six donors of COVID-19 vaccines.[108]

Serbia also tried its hand at vaccine diplomacy. The country ordered millions of doses of COVID-19 vaccines. With a vaccine-averse population and despite a high number of new cases, it wanted to earn goodwill and restore its past glory. Serbia decided to share the vaccines with its neighbouring countries.[109]

VACCINE DIPLOMACY: THE YEARS AHEAD

The COVID-19 pandemic has demonstrated the critical role played by vaccine diplomacy in decimating the deadly contagions. SARS-CoV-2 will continue to engulf lives and economies till herd immunity is reached and further mutations are stopped. This will not be possible until billions of people in resource-poor countries, desperately waiting in COVAX lines, are vaccinated.[46,51] This calls for strengthening of vaccine diplomacy.[88] The best way to fill the gap and avoid future epidemics is to do away with patent-related restrictions and support developing countries in manufacturing vaccines, both technically and financially.[46]

Accelerating the elimination of Neglected Tropical Diseases (NTDs) is another potential agenda of vaccine diplomacy. More than one billion people are affected annually by NTDs. However, vaccine development for NTDs is slow due to lack of a commercial market. One more challenge that can be addressed through vaccine diplomacy in the days to come is to increase vaccine coverage in areas of conflict and political instability.[110]

Countries need vaccine leaders to accomplish their goals, be it vaccination of their own population or using vaccines to secure diplomatic favours. The next chapter is dedicated to vaccine leaders, who have made victories against contagions possible.

REFERENCES

1. Katz R, Kornblet S, Arnold G, Lief E, Fischer JE. Defining health diplomacy: Changing demands in the era of globalization. *The Milbank Quarterly*. 2011 September;89(3):503–523.
2. Kickbusch I, Silberschmidt G, Buss P. Global health diplomacy: The need for new perspectives, strategic approaches and skills in global health. *Bulletin of the World Health Organization*. 2007;85: 230–232.
3. Afshari M, Teymourlouy AA, Asadi-Lari M, Maleki M. Global Health diplomacy for noncommunicable diseases prevention and control: A systematic review. *Globalization and Health*. 2020 Dec;16(1):1–6.
4. Alesina A, Dollar D. Who gives foreign aid to whom and why? *Journal of Economic Growth*. 2000 March;5(1):33–63.

5. Lee K, Smith R. Global health diplomacy: A conceptual review. *Global Health Governance*. 2011;5(1).
6. Hotez PJ. Vaccine diplomacy: Historical perspectives and future directions. *PLoS Neglected Tropical Diseases*. 2014 June;8(6):e2808.
7. Fidler DP. The globalization of public health: The first 100 years of international health diplomacy. *Bulletin of the World Health Organization*. 2001;79:842–849.
8. Gomez EJ. Cuba's health diplomacy in the age of Ebola. *BBC News*. November 2014.
9. Labonté R, Gagnon ML. Framing health and foreign policy: Lessons for global health diplomacy. *Globalization and Health*. 2010 December;6(1):1–9.
10. Fazal T M. Health diplomacy in pandemical times. *International Organization*. 2020 December;74(S1):E78–97.
11. Pandemic (H1N1) 2009 update 60. World Health Organization. Available from: https://www.who.int/csr/don/2009_08_04/en/
12. Tika Utsav and Vaccine Maitri: Finding the right balance [Internet]. Downtoearth.org.in. 2021 [cited 3 November 2021]. Available from: https://www.downtoearth.org.in/blog/health/tika-utsav-and-vaccine-maitri-finding-the-right-balance-76474
13. India's vaccine diplomacy. India China Institute [Internet]. India China Institute. 2021 [cited 3 November 2021]. Available from: https://www.indiachinainstitute.org/2021/03/04/indias_vaccine_diplomacy/#_ftn2
14. Singh SK. Global health diplomacy: A strategic opportunity for India. International Institute for Global Health. 2017.
15. Chaudhury DR. Covid diplomacy establishes India as a reliable and responsible global power. *The Economic Times*. 10 April 2020.
16. PM Modi asks G20 for an effective global response to coronavirus: Reports [Internet]. *Hindustan Times*. 2021 [cited 3 November 2021]. Available from: https://www.hindustantimes.com/india-news/pm-modi-asks-g20-for-an-effective-global-response-to-coronavirus-reports/story-myRgcYwmAhEX077ZZdGCbP.html
17. Pattanaik SS. COVID-19 Pandemic and India's Regional Diplomacy. *South Asian Survey*. 2021 March;28(1):92–110.
18. Surie M. India's COVID diplomacy. Development Policy Blog. [Internet]. 2021 [cited 3 November 2021]. Available from: https://devpolicy.org/indias-covid-diplomacy-20200603-2/
19. Arora N, Khanna S. India exports 50 million hydroxychloroquine tablets to US for COVID-19 fight. Reuters, April. 2020. 30.
20. Roche E. Covid-19 outbreak brings India's 'medical diplomacy' to world's notice [Internet]. *Mint*. 2021 [cited 3 November 2021]. Available from: https://www.livemint.com/news/india/covid-19-outbreak-brings-india-s-medical-diplomacy-to-world-s-notice-11587134032403.html
21. Roche E. Donald Trump all praise for India after deal on hydroxychloroquine [Internet]. *Mint*. 2021 [cited 3 November 2021]. Available from: https://

www.livemint.com/news/india/president-trump-full-of-praise-as-india-lifts-export-ban-on-hydroxychloroquine-11586318481567.html

22. City building through Indian Technical and Economic Cooperation (ITEC) [Internet]. Mea.gov.in. 2021 [cited 3 November 2021]. Available from: https://mea.gov.in/Portal/ForeignRelation/ITEC_new.pdf
23. Coronavirus. Prime Minister Modi calls for COVID-19 Emergency Fund for SAARC [Internet]. *The Hindu*. 2021 [cited 3 November 2021]. Available from: https://www.thehindu.com/news/national/coronavirus-pm-modi-participates-in-saarc-videoconference-to-formulate-joint-strategy-to-combat-covid-19/article31074653.ece
24. Economics of Influence: China and India in South Asia [Internet]. Council on Foreign Relations. 2021 [cited 3 November 2021]. Available from: https://www.cfr.org/expert-brief/economics-influence-china-and-india-south-asia
25. Banerjee A. India's flawed vaccine diplomacy. Stimson Center [Internet]. Stimson Center. 2021 [cited 3 November 2021]. Available from: https://www.stimson.org/2021/indias-flawed-vaccine-diplomacy/
26. Chan L H, L Chen, J Xu. China's engagement with global health diplomacy: Was SARS a watershed? Negotiating and navigating global health: Case studies in global health diplomacy 2012 (203–219).
27. Youde J. China's health diplomacy in Africa. *China: An International Journal*. 2010;8(1):151–63.
28. Lancaster K, Rubin M. Assessing the early response to Beijing's pandemic diplomacy. Council on Foreign Relations, 30 April 2020. Available from: https://www.cfr.org/blog/assessing-early-response-beijings-pandemic-diplomacy
29. Wu H, Gelineau K. China ships millions of COVID-19 vaccines to poor nations abroad; denies vaccine diplomacy. CP 24, 2 March 2021. Available from: https://www.cp24.com/world/china-ships-millions-of-covid-19-vaccines-to-poor-nations-abroad-denies-vaccine-diplomacy-1.5329782.
30. Burton G. China and COVID-19 in MENA. The COVID-19 pandemic in the Middle East and North Africa. 25 April 2020.
31. Bradsher K. China delays mask and ventilator exports after quality complaints. *The New York Times*. April 2020. 11:04.
32. China hopes 'vaccine diplomacy' will restore its image and boost its influence [Internet]. *The Guardian*. 2021 [cited 3 November 2021]. Available from: https://www.theguardian.com/world/2020/nov/29/china-hopes-vaccine-diplomacy-will-restore-its-image-and-boost-its-influence
33. Chatzky A, J McBride. China's massive belt and road initiative [Internet]. Council on Foreign Relations. 2021 [cited 3 November 2021]. Available from: https://www.cfr.org/backgrounder/chinas-massive-belt-and-road-initiative
34. Shakeel SI, Brown M, Sethi S, Mackey TK. Achieving the end game: Employing vaccine diplomacy to eradicate polio in Pakistan. *BMC Public Health*. 2019 December;19(1):1–8.
35. Pearson JD. Medical diplomacy and the American Indian: Thomas Jefferson, the Lewis and Clark Expedition and the subsequent effects

on American Indian health and public policy. *Wicazo Sa Review*. 2004 April;19(1):105–130.
36. Mihm S. Vaccines have united rival nations in the toughest of times [Internet]. Bloomberg.com. 2021 [cited 3 November 2021]. Available from: https://www.bloomberg.com/opinion/articles/2021-05-04/vaccine-diplomacy-in-history-smallpox-polio-covid-19
37. Pannu J, Barry M. The state inoculates: Vaccines as soft power. *The Lancet Global Health*. 2021 June;9(6):e744–745.
38. Hotez PJ. Peace through vaccine diplomacy. *Science*. 2010 March 12;327(5971):1301.
39. Vanderwagen W. Health diplomacy: winning hearts and minds through the use of health interventions. *Military Medicine*. 2006 October 1;171(10):3.
40. Varshney SK, Prasanna NK. Vaccine diplomacy: Exploring the benefits of international collaboration. Current Trends in Biotechnology and Pharmacy. 2021 February 12;5(1):110–114.
41. Novotny TE, Kickbusch I, Told M, editors. 21st century global health diplomacy. *World Scientific*. 13 June 2013.
42. Andrus JK, Ropero AM, Ghisays G, Romero S, Jauregui B, Matus CR. Yellow fever and health diplomacy: International efforts to stop the urban yellow fever outbreak in Paraguay. In: Rosskam E, Kickbusch I, editors *Negotiating And Navigating Global Health: Case Studies in Global Health Diplomacy*. Singapore: World Scientific Publishing Company; 2012. 391–403.
43. Kaufmann JR, Feldbaum H. Diplomacy and the polio immunization boycott in Northern Nigeria. *Health Affairs*. 2009 July;28(4):1091–1101.
44. Hotez PJ. Vaccines as instruments of foreign policy. *EMBO Reports*. 2001 October;2(10):862–868.
45. The US and Russia could join forces to get people vaccinated [Internet]. 2021 [cited 3 November 2021]. Available from: https://www.washingtonpost.com/outlook/2021/09/01/us-russia-could-join-forces-get-people-vaccinated-they-did-before/
46. Hotez PJ, Narayan KV. Restoring vaccine diplomacy. *JAMA*. 2021 May 28.
47. Rojansky M, Tabarovsky I. The latent power of health cooperation in US-Russian relations. *Science & Diplomacy*. 2013 June;2(2).
48. Hotez PJ. Russian–United States vaccine science diplomacy: Preserving the legacy. *PLoS Neglected Tropical Diseases*. 2017 May 25;11(5):e0005320.
49. Nye JS. Soft power. *Foreign Policy*. 1990 October;(80):153–171.
50. Rana V, Patel P, Mohyuddin S, Deb P. Vaccine Maitri: India faces a balancing act with its COVID-19 diplomacy. *LSE Business Review*. 26 April 2021.
51. Unmüßig B, Alexandra S. Divided we fail—vaccine diplomacy and its implications. Heinrich Böll Stiftung [Internet]. Heinrich-Böll-Stiftung. 2021 [cited 3 November 2021]. Available from: https://www.boell.de/en/2021/03/25/divided-we-fail-vaccine-diplomacy-and-its-implications

52. Israel secretly agrees to fund vaccines for Syria as part of prisoner swap [Internet]. Nytimes.com. 2021 [cited 3 November 2021]. Available from: https://www.nytimes.com/2021/02/20/world/middleeast/israel-syria-prisoner-swap-vaccines.html
53. Shepp J. The U.S. is playing catch-up at vaccine diplomacy [Internet]. Intelligencer. 2021 [cited 3 November 2021]. Available from: https://nymag.com/intelligencer/2021/05/the-u-s-is-playing-catch-up-at-vaccine-diplomacy.html
54. Taghizade S, Chattu VK, Jaafaripooyan E, Kevany S. COVID-19 pandemic as an excellent opportunity for Global Health Diplomacy. *Frontiers in Public Health*. 2021;9.
55. Twohey M, Collins K, Thomas K. With first dibs on vaccines, rich countries have 'cleared the shelves' [Internet]. Nytimes.com. 2021 [cited 3 November 2021]. Available from: https://www.nytimes.com/2020/12/15/us/coronavirus-vaccine-doses-reserved.html
56. PM's address at the 75th United Nations General Assembly (UNGA) session 2020 [Internet]. Pmindia.gov.in. 2021 [cited 3 November 2021]. Available from: https://www.pmindia.gov.in/en/news_updates/pms-address-at-the-75th-united-nations-general-assembly-unga-session-2020/?comment=disable&tag term=pmspeech
57. Chatterjee N, Mahmood Z, Marcussen E. Politics of vaccine nationalism in India: Global and domestic implications. *Forum for Development Studies*. 2021 May;48(2):1–13.
58. Reuters Staff. India to ship COVID-19 vaccines to Canada as diplomatic tension eases [Internet]. U.S. 2021 [cited 3 November 2021]. Available from: https://www.reuters.com/article/us-health-coronavirus-canada-idUSKBN2AF0KA
59. Chaulia S. Vaccine diplomacy is India's finest hour. Available from: http://dspace.jgu.edu.in:8080/jspui/bitstream/10739/4633/1/Vaccine%20diplomacy%20is%20Indias%20finest%20hour.pdf
60. Misra D. India's vaccine diplomacy: Able internationalism or abscondence of responsibility? *Pensamiento Propio*. 53:264.
61. Vaccine supply [Internet]. Mea.gov.in. 2021 [cited 3 November 2021]. Available from: https://www.mea.gov.in/vaccine-supply.htm
62. Sri Lanka orders 13.5 million AstraZeneca doses, likely to drop Chinese COVID-19 vaccines [Internet]. *The Hindu*. 2021 [cited 3 November 2021]. Available from: https://www.thehindu.com/news/international/sri-lanka-orders-135-million-astrazeneca-doses-likely-to-drop-chinese-covid-19-vaccines/article33913670.ece
63. Bose S. The dynamics of vaccine diplomacy in India's neighbourhood [Internet]. ORF. 2021 [cited 10 October 2021]. Available from: https://www.orfonline.org/research/the-dynamics-of-vaccine-diplomacy-in-indias-neighbourhood/

64. Government of India. Question No.3692 Neighbourhood First Policy. Media Centre, Ministry of External Affairs, 25 July 2019. Available from: https://mea.gov.in/rajya-sabha.htm?dtl/31673/QUESTION+NO3692+NEIGHBOURHOOD+FIRST+POLICY
65. Worldview with Suhasini Haidar: What went wrong with India's vaccine diplomacy? [Internet]. *The Hindu*. 2021 [cited 10 October 2021]. Available from: https://www.thehindu.com/news/national/worldview-with-suhasini-haidar-what-went-wrong-with-indias-vaccine-diplomacy/article34394622.ece
66. Bhardwaj S. Made in Hyderabad vaccine key weapon in Quad arsenal to counter China | Hyderabad News. *Times of India* [Internet]. *Times of India*. 2021 [cited 3 November 2021]. Available from: https://timesofindia.indiatimes.com/city/hyderabad/made-in-hyd-vax-key-weapon-in-quad-arsenal-to-counter-china/articleshow/81488679.cms
67. Chaudhury D. India set to produce coronavirus vaccine under Quad initiative with US, Japan and Australia [Internet]. *The Economic Times*. 2021 [cited 3 November 2021]. Available from: https://economictimes.indiatimes.com/news/politics-and-nation/india-set-to-produce-coronavirus-vaccine-under-quad-initiative-with-us-japan-and-australia/articleshow/81477642.cms
68. Vinayak A. Vaccine Maitri: A sanjeevini for the world [Internet]. @businessline. 2021 [cited 3 November 2021]. Available from: https://www.thehindubusinessline.com/news/variety/vaccine-maitri-a-sanjeevini-for-the-world/article33989241.ece
69. Manral K. Bill Gates hails India's leadership in scientific innovation, vaccine manufacturing [Internet]. *Hindustan Times*. 2021 [cited 3 November 2021]. Available from: https://www.hindustantimes.com/world-news/bill-gates-hails-india-s-leadership-in-scientific-innovation-vaccine-manufacturing/story-9k9Cn7yiTzssG5es5eKKrJ.html
70. Dhume S. Opinion. India Beats China at Vaccine Diplomacy [Internet]. WSJ. 2021 [cited 3 November 2021]. Available from: https://www.wsj.com/articles/india-beats-china-at-vaccine-diplomacy-11616086729
71. IANS. India, a vaccine hub for the world! 92 countries request for stock [Internet]. Indiatvnews.com. 2021 [cited 3 November 2021]. Available from: https://www.indiatvnews.com/news/india/india-made-vaccines-in-demand-92-countries-request-order-serum-institute-Covishield-Covaxin-latest-news-679537
72. US 'applauds' India for gifting Covid-19 vaccine to several countries [Internet]. *Mint*. 2021 [cited 3 November 2021]. Available from: https://www.livemint.com/news/world/us-applauds-india-for-gifting-covid-19-vaccine-to-several-countries-11611368801097.html
73. Delhi pushes ahead with vaccine diplomacy as Indian supplies on top demand [Internet]. *The Federal*. 2021 [cited 3 November 2021]. Available from: https://thefederal.com/covid-19/delhi-pushes-ahead-with-vaccine-diplomacy-as-indian-supplies-on-top-demand/

74. Chawla D. Diplomacy in difficult times: India's Vaccine Maitri initiative. [Internet]. Investindia.gov.in. 2021 [cited 3 November 2021]. Available from: https://www.investindia.gov.in/team-india-blogs/diplomacy-difficult-times-indias-vaccine-maitri-initiative
75. Bery A. Vaccine diplomacy: Advantage India [Internet]. *South Asian Voices*. 2021 [cited 3 November 2021]. Available from: https://southasianvoices.org/vaccine-diplomacy-advantage-india/
76. US Congressman praises India for supplying Covid-19 vaccines to neighbours. *Global Partners* [Internet]. News18. 2021 [cited 3 November 2021]. Available from: https://www.news18.com/news/world/us-congressman-praises-india-for-supplying-covid-19-vaccines-to-neighbours-global-partners-3290219.html
77. India's reputation as pharmacy of world reinforced; made-in-India vaccines supplied to 72 nations. Jaishankar [Internet]. *The Economic Times*. 2021 [cited 3 November 2021]. Available from: https://economictimes.indiatimes.com/news/politics-and-nation/indias-reputation-as-pharmacy-of-world-reinforced-made-in-india-vaccines-supplied-to-72-nations-jaishankar/articleshow/81550415.cms?from=mdr
78. Tharoor S. India's smart vaccine diplomacy by Shashi Tharoor—Project Syndicate [Internet]. Project Syndicate. 2021 [cited 3 November 2021]. Available from: https://www.project-syndicate.org/commentary/india covid19-vaccine-diplomacy-by-shashi-tharoor-2021 03
79. Bimal S. Time for India to reinvigorate vaccine diplomacy in South Asia [Internet]. *The Wire*. 2021 [cited 3 November 2021]. Available from: https://thewire.in/trade/time-for-india-to-reinvigorate-vaccine-diplomacy-in-south-asia
80. Kumar C. Covid-19 vaccine India: Each vaccine vial, with 10 doses, must be used within 4 hours of opening. India News. *Times of India* [Internet]. *Times of India*. 2021 [cited 3 November 2021]. Available from: https://timesofindia.indiatimes.com/india/each-vaccine-vial-with-10-doses-must-be-used-within-4-hours-of-opening/articleshow/80205276.cms
81. Yang S. Rising-power competition: The Covid-19 vaccine diplomacy of China and India. *Emerging Voices on the New Normal in Asia, National Bureau of Asian Research*. 2021 March;19:2.
82. Jennings R. China's COVID-19 vaccine diplomacy reaches 100-plus countries [Internet]. VOA. 2021 [cited 3 November 2021]. Available from: https://www.voanews.com/a/china-s-covid-19-vaccine-diplomacy-reaches-100-plus-countries/6233766.html
83. Voss G, Zhou J, Shuldiner H. Vaccine diplomacy in Latin America [Internet]. Wilson Center. 2021 [cited 3 November 2021]. Available from: https://www.wilsoncenter.org/blog-post/vaccine-diplomacy-latin-america
84. Sui-Lee W. China wanted to show off its vaccines. It's backfiring. [Internet]. Nytimes.com. 2021 [cited 3 November 2021]. Available from: https://www.nytimes.com/2021/01/25/business/china-covid-19-vaccine-backlash.html

85. Yen NL. [Internet]. 2021 [cited 3 November 2021]. Available from: https://www.cnbc.com/2021/06/10/covid-expert-on-us-china-competition-in-vaccine-diplomacy.html
86. Is China's vaccine success fading in Asia? [Internet]. *The ASEAN Post*. 2021 [cited 3 November 2021]. Available from: https://theaseanpost.com/article/chinas-vaccine-success-fading-asia
87. UAE has sufficient vaccine supplies to support need for third 'booster' dose, health expert says [Internet]. 2021 [cited 3 November 2021]. Available from: https://www.thenationalnews.com/uae/health/uae-has-sufficient-vaccine-supplies-to-support-need-for-third-booster-dose-health-expert-says-1.1188560
88. Aspinall E. The rise of vaccine diplomacy. British Foreign Policy Group [Internet]. British Foreign Policy Group. 2021 [cited 3 November 2021]. Available from: https://bfpg.co.uk/2021/07/the-rise-of-vaccine-diplomacy/
89. Hasan M. China is using vaccines to extend its influence in Asia [Internet]. MarshMcLennan. Conversations and Insights on Global Business. 2021 [cited 3 November 2021]. Available from: https://www.brinknews.com/china-is-using-vaccines-to-extend-its-influence-in-asia/
90. Basu N. Modi govt plans to revive 'Vaccine Maitri' in July-August, but only in neighbourhood [Internet]. 2021 [cited 3 November 2021]. Available from: https://theprint.in/diplomacy/modi-govt-plans-to-revive-vaccine-maitri-in-july-august-but-only-in-neighbourhood/682758/
91. Grossman D. What China wants in South Asia. 2020 October;26:2020. Available from: https://www.orfonline.org/research/what-china-wants-in-south-asia-67665/
92. Krishnan A. Bangladesh rebuffs China on Quad warning. *The Hindu*. Available from: https://www.thehindu.com/news/international/bangladesh-rebuffs-china-on-quad-warning/article34542373.ece
93. Mitra D. With none of the earlier fanfare in sight, India resumes COVID-19 vaccine exports [Internet]. *The Wire*. 2022 [cited 18 January 2022]. Available from: https://thewire.in/diplomacy/india-covid-19-vaccine-maitri-branding
94. India's offer of South Asian response to COVID-19 counter to China's attempts to change narrative [Internet]. *The Economic Times*. 2021 [cited 3 November 2021]. Available from: https://economictimes.indiatimes.com/news/politics-and-nation/indias-offer-of-south-asian-response-to-covid-19-counter-to-chinas-attempts-to-change-narrative/articleshow/74983341.cms?from=mdr
95. Gupta S. Dhaka turned to India for vaccine after China wanted Bangladesh to share clinical trials' cost [Internet]. *Hindustan Times*. 2021 [cited 3 November 2021]. Available from: https://www.hindustantimes.com/india-news/how-dhaka-got-vaccines-from-india-after-china-asked-it-to-share-trial-costs-101611459036601-amp.html
96. Blablová V. How China and India are competing in vaccine diplomacy [Internet]. *chinaobservers*. 2021 [cited 3 November 2021]. Available

from: https://chinaobservers.eu/how-china-and-india-are-competing-in-vaccine-diplomacy/
97. Staff R. Vaccine refusal in Brazil grows to 22%, most reject Chinese shot: Poll [Internet]. U.S. 2021 [cited 3 November 2021]. Available from: https://www.reuters.com/article/us-health-coronavirus-brazil-idUSKBN28M0VC
98. Ramani S. With Sputnik V, Russia shot itself in the foot [Internet]. Foreign Policy. 2021 [cited 3 November 2021]. Available from: https://foreignpolicy.com/2021/06/24/russia-sputnik-v-vaccine-diplomacy-africa-prices-delays/
99. Bautzer T, Boadle A. Brazil maker of Sputnik V vaccine sees green light on tests by next week [Internet]. U.S. 2021 [cited 3 November 2021]. Available from: https://www.reuters.com/article/us-health-coronavirus-brazil-sputnik-idUSKBN2A22OI
100. Stronski P, Kier G. Russia's vaccine diplomacy is mostly smoke and mirrors [Internet]. Carnegie Endowment for International Peace. 2021 [cited 3 November 2021]. Available from: https://carnegieendowment.org/2021/08/03/russia-s-vaccine-diplomacy-is-mostly-smoke-and-mirrors-pub-85074
101. Kriminger T. Vaccine diplomacy dilemma: A double-edged sword? Atlas Institute for International Affairs [Internet]. Atlas Institute for International Affairs. 2021 [cited 9 October 2021]. Available from: https://www.internationalaffairshouse.org/the-vaccine-diplomacy-dilemma-a-double-edged-sword/
102. Reality Check team. Coronavirus G7: Could a billion more vaccines for poorer countries make a difference? [Internet]. *BBC News*. 2021 [cited 3 November 2021]. Available from: https://www.bbc.com/news/57427877
103. Mason J, O'donnell C. Under pressure, U.S. donates half billion more COVID-19 vaccine doses to world [Internet]. Reuters. 2021 [cited 3 November 2021]. Available from: https://www.reuters.com/world/us/biden-pledges-new-vaccine-donations-bid-rally-global-pandemic-fight-2021-09-22/
104. Japan's COVID-19-related cooperation [Internet]. Mofa.go.jp. 2021 [cited 3 November 2021]. Available from: https://www.mofa.go.jp/files/100231344.pdf
105. Japan stepping up vaccine diplomacy to counter Chinese influence [Internet]. *The Japan Times*. 2021 [cited 3 November 2021]. Available from: https://www.japantimes.co.jp/news/2021/06/19/national/japan-vaccine-diplomacy/
106. Galeeva D. Small states response to Covid-19: View from the UAE. *Project on Middle East Political Science (POMEPS)*. 2020 April;39:38–40. Available from: https://pomeps.org/wp-content/uploads/2020/04/POMEPS_Studies_39_Web.pdf
107. Soubrier E. Gulf humanitarian diplomacy in the time of coronavirus. Arab Gulf States Institute Washington; 1 May 2020. Available from: https://agsiw.org/gulf-humanitarian-diplomacy-in-the-time-of-coronavirus/

108. Alexander K, Mazzucco LJ. Insight 261: Vaccine diplomacy–UAE tries to balance hard times with soft power. Available from: https://mei.nus.edu.sg/publication/insight-261-vaccine-diplomacy-the-uae-tries-to-balance-hard-times-with-soft-power/
109. Hopkins V. Bounty of Serbian vaccine diplomacy shames the EU [Internet]. Ft.com. 2021 [cited 3 November 2021]. Available from: https://www.ft.com/content/81fc28aa-04a9-4108-a69b-80dc93a9e985
110. Hotez PJ. Immunizations and vaccines: A decade of successes and reversals, and a call for vaccine diplomacy. *International Health*. 2019 September 2;11(5):331–333.

Chapter 9

Promoting Mass Vaccinations: Role of Leadership

Vaccines have enabled humanity to conquer many pernicious contagions. However, apart from discovery of vaccines, strong leadership is needed to enable mass vaccination in order to triumph over virulent diseases.

WHY IS LEADERSHIP CRITICAL FOR MASS VACCINATION?

Although the development of a vaccine is an extraordinary achievement, mere approval and rollout of the vaccine does not end an infectious disease. Effective protection requires herd immunity, which can only be achieved by mass vaccination. Apart from arranging for mass vaccination, convincing people to take the shots is a difficult task that needs effective leaders at various levels.[1]

Leadership is the process of social influence wherein one person mobilizes the support of others to accomplish a common task.[2] Therefore, aside from the technical aspects and interpersonal relationships, leadership in mass vaccination programmes needs conceptual and effective communication skills.[3] Leadership implies a number of people leading at different times and in varying ways.[2] This is true for vaccination-related leadership as well and extends from the global to the grassroot level.[4]

POLITICAL LEADERSHIP: A CATALYST TO CONVINCE PEOPLE

Since the time of variolation, political leadership has played a critical role in conveying the gravity of the problem caused by infectious diseases, the significance of vaccination in decimating them and mobilizing people to opt for inoculation.[5] History has numerous such examples to offer.

EMPEROR K'ANG-HSI: SMALLPOX GIFTS THE THRONE

K'ang-hsi ascended the throne in China in the late 1600s, courtesy smallpox. As the third son, he had no chance of becoming the emperor. But when his father succumbed to smallpox at the young age of 23, the pockmarked K'ang-hsi was chosen over his elder brothers to succeed him because he had survived the smallpox pandemic.

The new emperor became a strong supporter of variolation. K'ang-hsi inoculated his children, troops and people. His efforts and personal example popularized inoculation in China and saved precious lives. To motivate future generations to carry on this practice, K'ang-hsi wrote a letter to his descendants explaining the impact of what he had done and that he was proud of his achievement.[6]

CAROLINE OF ANSBACH: FACILITATOR OF FIRST CLINICAL TRIAL

Caroline of Ansbach, the Princess of Wales, was another leader who promoted inoculations. With her assistance, what may be called the first clinical trial was conducted on seven condemned prisoners of Newgate Prison in London in August 1721. All of them survived. This was followed by testing the efficacy of inoculation on orphan children in Westminster.[7,8]

Following the success of the two trials, Caroline got her three children, Amelia, Caroline and Frederic, inoculated in April 1722. Although her motives were not completely altruistic, inoculation of the royal children without ill-effects led to widespread acceptance of variolation.[9,10]

CATHERINE THE GREAT: SECRET INOCULATION

In 1768, Catherine the Great of Russia got herself and her son, the future Tsar of Russia, inoculated. She became the first person to be inoculated against smallpox in Russia. Catherine invited physician Thomas Dimsdale from England for the variolation. This was kept a closely guarded secret. There were relays of horses deployed in complete readiness to facilitate Dimsdale's escape from angry Russians in case the inoculation went wrong.[11]

Catherine recovered and became a champion of inoculation. She organized inoculation drives and urged her subjects to be vaccinated. She issued detailed instructions to authorities on how they should organize inoculation campaigns.[11]

GEORGE WASHINGTON: INOCULATIONS TO SAVE THE REVOLUTION

In late 1776, George Washington was leading the opening battles of the American Revolution. However, his troops were facing the biggest threat not from the enemy but from Variola. A smallpox outbreak had already led to their defeat in the Battle of Quebec. Smallpox not only deterred enrolment in the army but also posed the risk of debilitating his troops.[12]

Washington ordered mass inoculation of his men.[12] Variolation started on 6 February 1777, and by the end of the year, more than 40,000 soldiers had been inoculated.[13,14] The vaccines turned out to be a critically important in the eventual outcome of the War of Independence and saved the revolution.[15,16]

THOMAS JEFFERSON: VACCINATING THE AMERICAN PEOPLE

Thomas Jefferson, the third President of the USA, was one of the early advocates of smallpox vaccination. He followed the work of Edward Jenner and supported the introduction of the cowpox vaccine to America.

Jefferson worked with Benjamin Waterhouse, an American physician. Jefferson declared smallpox vaccination a national public health priority. He assisted Waterhouse by providing physicians and vaccines from England. He also invited Native American tribal leaders to Washington to demonstrate inoculation.[17,18]

KING CARLOS IV: THE VACCINE CRUSADER

Jenner's discovery of the smallpox vaccine needed mass vaccination leaders to use it to eradicate the scourge. One of the pioneers was King Carlos IV of Spain. Carlos decided to protect the people in his colonies from smallpox. Therefore, in 1803, he launched an expedition led by the Royal Surgeon, Francisco Javier de Balmis.[19]

King Carlos issued a royal order on 1 September 1803 to all officers and religious authorities in his domains, informing them of the arrival of the Balmis expedition and directing them to support vaccination of the masses.[19,20]

Balmis took the vaccine lymph to America and Asia by conducting arm-to-arm vaccinations of foundlings. For this, 22 children aged 3–9 years from the Santiago de Compostela orphanage were selected.[21,22]

PROFESSOR VIKTOR ZHDANOV: CONVINCING THE WORLD THAT IT CAN DEFEAT SMALLPOX

An important name in the history of global vaccine leadership is Viktor Mikhailovich Zhdanov. He was a Soviet virologist and epidemiologist. In 1958, when Zhdanov was the USSR's Deputy

Minister of Health, he brought a resolution to the World Health Assembly proposing a 10-year campaign to eradicate smallpox.

Zhdanov promised 25 million vaccines to initiate the programme and offered a technique known as lyophilization, or freeze-drying, of the vaccine. Zhdanov's arguments convinced the World Health Assembly, which accepted the 'Zhdanov resolution'. A global campaign for the eradication of smallpox followed in 1959.

FRANKLIN ROOSEVELT: MOVER OF THE 'MARCH OF DIMES'

Polio was another scourge that has been almost decimated by vaccination leaders. A prominent political name in polio vaccination leadership is of the US President Franklin Delano Roosevelt. Both his legs were paralysed by polio in August 1921.[23]

The costs associated with polio research were high and research funding was scarce. Roosevelt supported research through fundraisers on his birthday, starting from 1934.[23] In 1938, he founded the National Foundation for Infantile Paralysis.

Roosevelt became the icon of the 'March of Dimes', a grassroot fundraising campaign. It exhorted people to send dimes for polio research to the President.[8] The campaign raised millions of dollars. It supported both Jonas Salk's inactivated vaccine and Sabin's OPV.[17,24]

DEFEATING THE TWO DEMONS: THE INDIAN SUCCESS STORY

Despite all odds, India has been able to eradicate two of the greatest scourges: smallpox and polio. Let us see how.

India Eradicates Variola

India has borne the maximum brunt of smallpox. In 1963, it reported more than 80 per cent of all known cases and 75 per cent of all deaths from smallpox globally.[25]

To eradicate the disease, the Indian government launched its National Smallpox Eradication Programme (NSEP) in 1962. Its aim was mass vaccination, but it failed to defeat the contagion. The programme was reoriented in 1973 and focused on surveillance and containment. The then Prime Minister, Mrs Indira Gandhi, threw her weight behind the programme.[26,27]

Many were concealing the disease due to fear of stigma and social isolation. Therefore, beginning in June 1973, a nationwide house-to-house manhunt for the smallpox virus was launched. A total of two billion house calls were made.[28] A reward of ₹100 was announced for reporting a case of smallpox. It was later increased to ₹1,000.[29]

The last case of smallpox was reported in India on 17 May 1975. In the last week of April 1977, the WHO declared India free of the deadly scourge.

India's Fight against Polio

Due to its huge and diverse population, unhygienic conditions in the country and other challenges, people doubted India's ability to eradicate polio. However, starting in the mid-90s, a new approach and effective leadership ensured that polio was eradicated from the country.

In 1994, pulse polio immunization was initiated in Tamil Nadu with grants provided by Rotary International. On 2 October 1994, it was expanded to Kerala and Delhi.[30] A national roll out of the vaccine followed in July 1995. India accounted for around 60 per cent of polio cases worldwide at that time.[30]

With the tagline 'Do Boond Zindagi Ki' (two drops of life), the programme raised awareness about polio and its vaccination. The initiative roped in celebrities, including film stars and cricketers.

Irrespective of the party in power, immunization efforts continued year after year. Starting in 2004, annual pulse polio vaccination campaigns were carried out 10 times a year. Every child was tracked and vaccinated.

Apart from ensuring equitable access to vaccines, the government simultaneously addressed social and cultural concerns to remove vaccine hesitancy. The last polio cases were reported in India in 2011. In 2014, India was officially declared polio-free.[31,32,33]

NARENDRA MODI: THE MAN BEHIND THE WORLD'S LARGEST VACCINATION DRIVE

COVID-19 was a huge crisis in which the Indian Prime Minister, Narendra Modi, emerged as a decisive vaccination leader. Apart from providing funds for vaccine development, he encouraged vaccine manufacturers through regular interactions. He also visited their manufacturing facilities in Ahmedabad, Hyderabad and Pune.[34]

Modi supported vaccine development and eased regulatory approvals. 'The Prime Minister went out of his way and made all the regulatory people move very fast,' said Cyrus Poonawalla, the head of SII, the world's largest vaccine manufacturer.[35]

Apart from launching the world's largest vaccine drive in India, Narendra Modi enabled many developing countries to start their COVID-19 vaccination drives. From the beginning, he made it clear that India stands in solidarity with the world. 'India will make available its vaccine-manufacturing prowess to the entire world in the spirit of *Vasudhaiv Kutumbkam*,' he told the UN General Assembly in September 2020. India also worked with its QUAD partners to meet the global demand for COVID-19 vaccines.[36]

Modi's leadership made the world's largest vaccination drive undertaken by India a resounding success. In the initial phases of the drive, when vaccine hesitancy was high, he promoted vaccination by launching Teeka Utsav across India in April 2020. Later, when the second wave of the COVID-19 pandemic struck, there was a mad rush for vaccines. The prime minister ensured that top political and bureaucratic functionaries did not jump the queue.

On 21 October 2021, India made history by crossing the milestone of one billion (100 crore) vaccinations against COVID-19. The Union Health Secretary, Rajesh Bhushan, while talking to me, acknowledged that the milestone could only be achieved due to political leadership and commitment at the highest level. 'The Hon'ble Prime Minister, Shri Narendra Modi Ji, led the national COVID-19 vaccination effort from the front', he said.

However, the Prime Minister Modi ensured that there was no complacency. He told officials that 'diseases and enemies should be fought against till the very end'.[37] He asked them to change gears and go door-to-door to administer the COVID-19 vaccination. He also gave them the mantra: 'Har Ghar Tika, Ghar Tika' (vaccine at every doorstep) and 'Har Ghar Dastak' (knocking on every door) to reach every household.[38]

INDIVIDUAL LEADERS

Many individuals showed exemplary leadership in the fight against infectious diseases when it came to mass vaccination.

Lady Mary Wortley Montagu: Taking Variolation to Royalty

Lady Montague introduced variolation to Britain. She had witnessed this practice in March 1717 in Constantinople, where her husband was the ambassador of Britain. Seeing the effectiveness of the process, she asked the Embassy surgeon, Charles Maitland, to inoculate her five-year-old son, Edward.

On returning to London, she worked hard to popularize the procedure, despite stiff resistance from the English medical community. Montagu decided to get her daughter inoculated. She invited physicians and prominent people to witness the procedure.

After her daughter's recovery, Montagu took her to the houses of smallpox patients to demonstrate the efficacy of variolation. Montagu's efforts convinced Caroline of Ansbach, the Princess of Wales, to inoculate her children.

Rev. Cotton Mather: Inoculator Undeterred by Bombs

Rev. Cotton Mather was an influential Puritan minister in New England. Despite stiff opposition, Mather introduced and popularized variolation in the USA.[8]

The smallpox epidemic struck Boston in the spring of 1721. As the epidemic worsened, Mather reached out to Boston's medical community, pleading with them to inoculate people. Only one physician, Zabdiel Boylston, agreed. Others were hostile to the idea.

Boylston personally variolated 287 people. Only 2 per cent of them died, compared to 14.8 per cent of those who had contracted the disease naturally.[39] However, Boylson and Mather were accused of infecting people with a 'negroish disease'. In November 1921, a bomb was hurled at Mather's house. Boylston was assaulted in the streets and his house was also attacked.[39]

Dr William H. Foege: The Ring Vaccinator

While working in eastern Nigeria in 1967, Dr Foege demonstrated that vaccination of people (rather than whole populations) who could have been exposed to the smallpox virus could stop transmission. His technique was called 'ring vaccination'.

Ring vaccination entailed rapid reporting of cases and prompt vaccination of the family members and close contacts of confirmed cases. It soon became a part of the worldwide vaccination campaign.

Foege also made huge efforts to increase immunization rates in developing countries. In 1973, on the request of the WHO, the CDC loaned Foege to tackle smallpox in India. He persuaded the Indian Government not to reduce its commitment to smallpox eradication.[27] He also suggested that the Indian Government should institute a reward system to overcome people's resistance to reporting cases.

Donald A. Henderson

Donald Ainslie Henderson, an American epidemiologist, played a key leadership role in decimating smallpox. As the Chief of the Centers for Disease Control and Prevention(CDC) virus disease surveillance programme from 1960 to 1965, Henderson worked tirelessly to eliminate smallpox and control measles through vaccination. This initiative gave an impetus to the WHO's programme to eradicate smallpox.

In 1966 Henderson was appointed the head of the WHO's global smallpox eradication campaign.[40] He was a fierce supporter of field workers who marched tirelessly across the world until the last natural case of smallpox was diagnosed on 26 October 1977.[41]

In 1974, Henderson orchestrated the WHO's Expanded Program on Immunization (EPI). This initiative led to vaccination of 80 per cent of the world's children against six major diseases.[42]

Dr Tedros Adhanom Ghebreyesus: A Champion of Vaccine Equity

Dr Tedros Adhanom Ghebreyesus is a dedicated, charismatic and brilliant mass vaccination leader. He was elected the Director-General of the WHO in May 2017. The first test of his leadership came immediately when an Ebola outbreak was reported in the Democratic Republic of Congo. Leading the response from the front, Dr Tedros visited the country multiple times at great personal risk. He enthused the health workers who worked hard and vaccinated over 300,000 people amidst active conflict.

His next challenge, the pandemic of the century, knocked on doors soon. The WHO, under Tedros, launched the ACT Accelerator to speed up development of medicines, diagnostics and vaccines[43] As early as August 2020, Dr Tedros declared that the main mission of the WHO was to marshal global vaccine candidates through clinical trials, followed by fair and equitable availability of vaccines. To achieve this objective, the WHO under his leadership, unveiled the COVAX facility on 21 September 2020.

As the vaccine was rolled out, Dr Tedros spoke forcefully and repeatedly for vaccine equity and against the global disparity in distribution of COVID-19 vaccines. He labelled vaccine inequity as 'vaccine apartheid' and a 'catastrophic moral failure'.[44] He appealed to countries and vaccine manufacturers to ensure that more vaccines were available and provided to states that were not wealthy.

Although Dr Tedros was maligned, abused, vilified with a racist slur and threatened, he rose above all obstacles to focus on mass vaccination for COVID-19. The success of his leadership in handling the pandemic and mass vaccination was demonstrated by his re-endorsement for a second term as the Director General of the WHO, unchallenged.[45]

SCIENTIST LEADERS

Many scientists not only discovered vaccines against infectious diseases but also played a key role in promoting their production of vaccines and mass vaccination.

Edward Jenner: World's Vaccine Clerk

Dr Edward Jenner, who discovered the smallpox vaccine, ushered in a new era in the fight against infectious diseases.[46,47] He decided to spend the rest of his life encouraging physicians to vaccinate people and supplying them with the cowpox vaccine.

Due to Jenner's concerted efforts, smallpox vaccines reached many countries. Since Jenner was 'drowned' in correspondence about his vaccine, he called himself 'the vaccine clerk of the world'. Apart from the vaccine, Jenner also developed techniques for quick and wide transport of cowpox matter.[48]

Dr Benjamin Waterhouse: The Jenner of America

Dr Benjamin Waterhouse, a Harvard professor, took Jenner's discovery to the 'New World'. He corresponded with Jenner and received from him some threads that were impregnated with the vaccine matter. On 8 July 1800, he performed the first vaccination in the USA.

Dr Waterhouse decided to write to John Adams, the then President of the USA, requesting him to promote vaccination. When he failed to get a response, he wrote to the Vice President, Thomas Jefferson, who responded and offered his support.

Initially, Dr Waterhouse thought of monopolizing vaccination and aimed to make profit.[49] However, soon he became a major advocate of free vaccination and distributed the vaccine matter free of cost to physicians along with printed instructions on vaccination.[50]

He conducted a public trial of vaccination for Boston's Board of Health. On 16 August 1802, he vaccinated 19 boys and later exposed them to the smallpox virus. The success of the trial led the board to urge the public to take advantage of the procedure.[51]

Ernest Chambon: The Vaccine Cultivator

For almost several decades, arm-to-arm vaccination was the only way known to the world to disseminate and maintain the smallpox vaccine. In the middle of the 19th century, Giuseppe Negri succeeded in producing a vaccine in calves in Naples in Italy. However, the man who first started mass production of an 'animal vaccine' was Ernest Chambon.

In 1860, Chambon, then a medical student, attended a Medical Congress in Lyon in France where the animal vaccine was discussed. Chambon realized its potential and convinced his friend

Gustave Lanoix to visit Naples to learn the technique from Negri. Lanoix obliged and returned to Paris with a vaccinated heifer. The vaccine material from the heifer was grown by serial propagation in calves. Chambon and Lanoix set up a private vaccine production facility named, the Institute of Animal Vaccines, in Paris in 1864.[52,53]

The animal vaccine had many advantages. It insured a constant supply of the vaccine, enabled its production in large quantities and provided people protection from transmission of syphilis and other human diseases.[52] Chambon and Lanoix's concept spread across the world quickly.[52]

Luis Pasteur: Progenitor of Immunology

Luis Pasteur, the famous French biologist, microbiologist and chemist, is regarded as the father of immunology. He discovered vaccines for chicken cholera, anthrax and rabies. This tireless and dedicated scientist found that germs causing diseases can be weakened by exposing them to adverse environmental conditions or passing them repetitively through animals of a different species. When administered in the body, these attenuated germs would cause a mild ailment that would make the recipient immune to the stronger version of the disease. As a tribute to Jenner, he called this weak form of the pathogen 'vaccine'.[54]

Through the rabies vaccine, Pasteur demonstrated that if a person is vaccinated soon enough after infection, this can prevent disease and death.[55] He produced the first laboratory vaccine, which ushered in a revolution for mass production of vaccines.[8]

Waldemar Haffkine: The Saviour of Humanity

Waldemar Haffkine developed the first vaccine against a human bacterial disease. He discovered vaccines for cholera and plague.[56]

Haffkine had developed an anti-cholera vaccine at the Pasteur Institute in Paris in 1892. However, he needed to test it on a larger population. This brought him to India in 1893.[57]

Haffkine spent hours inoculating people every day with the cholera vaccine. These included slum dwellers, tea garden workers, army troops and others.[57,58] The success of his vaccine among the Indian population was phenomenal. By 1900, Haffkine had saved four million people.[59]

Haffkine's next challenge was bubonic plague, which had reached Bombay in September 1896. The Governor requested Haffkine to help to control the disease. He was ready with a killed vaccine for plague in January 1897.

Haffkine conducted a trial of his plague vaccine on the inmates of Bombay's Byculla Jail.[58,60,61] It was a resounding success and set the stage for mass vaccination. Within a year, thousands of people were inoculated with Haffkine's vaccine.[61]

Jonas Salk: The Miracle Worker

The next big revolution in mass vaccination was ushered in by Jonas Edward Salk, a US virologist. He was hailed as a miracle worker. Salk developed the first successful vaccine against polio. It was a 'killed' virus vaccine.[62]

The vaccine was tested on one million children in 1954. Mass vaccination started in 1955 and the average number of cases in the USA dropped from 45,000 annually to just 910 in 1962.[63] By 1959, Salk's vaccine had reached around 90 countries.[64]

Salk believed that public health was a 'moral commitment' and campaigned for mandatory vaccination.[65] To ensure that the vaccine reached the largest number of children, he refused to patent his vaccine. To commemorate this vaccination leader, the world celebrates World Polio Day on 24 October every year.[63,66]

Albert Sabin: The Poliomyelitis Terminator

The US scientist Dr Albert Sabin successfully grew the poliomyelitis virus in brain tissue taken from a human embryo in 1936. After growing and testing several strains of the virus, Sabin found three mutant strains of poliovirus that stimulated an immune response without causing paralysis. Using these attenuated strains, he developed a trivalent oral vaccine.[65]

However, Sabin was unable to secure adequate support for large-scale field trials of his vaccine, as Salk's vaccine was being used successfully in the USA. Therefore, in 1957, he approached the Soviet Union for field studies of his vaccine. The trials were successfully concluded on 10 million Soviet children. The vaccine was approved for commercial use in 1961. Soon Sabin's vaccine became the world's weapon against polio.[64] Like Jonas Salk, Albert Sabin did not patent his vaccine.

WOMEN'S VACCINATION LEADERSHIP

The story of vaccines is incomplete without a mention of the women leaders who worked tirelessly against all odds to defeat diseases. At the grassroot level, women contribute 70 per cent to the global health workforce and have played a lead role in mass vaccination.

Women have made a vital contribution to the development of vaccines and to disseminating their benefits. Even before the discovery of the smallpox vaccine, we know that many women leaders such as Caroline of Ansbach, Catherine the Great and Lady Mary Wortley Montagu had popularized variolation.

In the post-Jenner era, Dr Anna Wessels Williams contributed to the development of the diphtheria vaccine by isolating a high-yielding strain and also developing a rabies vaccine. Dr Pearl Kendrick and Dr Grace Eldering developed a vaccine for whooping cough, Dr Margaret Pittman's work led to the development of the first haemophilus influenzae vaccine[67] and Dr Isabel Morgan's work prepared a solid basis for the development of Jonas Salk's polio vaccine. Dr Anne Szarewski's work helped in development of the HPV vaccine; Professor Ruth Frances Bishop led the discovery of rotavirus; Rachel Schneerson pioneered the development of the first conjugate vaccine for haemophilus influenza[68]; Dr Gagandeep Kang developed India's first indigenous vaccine for rotavirus.[69]

Women leaders have also played a key role in overcoming COVID-19. There are many women leaders who have contributed actively to the development of COVID-19 vaccines at a breath-taking pace.[70]

India's first indigenous vaccine, COVAXIN, saw the light of day due to the untiring efforts of Dr K Sumathy at Bharat Biotech. Another Indian scientist, Dr Nita Patel, led an all-woman team at Novavax for vaccine development. The Oxford AstraZeneca vaccine owes its development to Professor Sarah Gilbert at the Oxford Vaccine Centre.[70] Another pioneer, Katalin Karikó, co-developed the mRNA technology that is used to produce the COVID-19 vaccines made by Pfizer and Moderna.

Özlem Türeci, a German immunologist and co-founder of BioNTech, worked round the clock to develop the company's COVID-19 vaccine; Dr Kizzmekia Corbett led the researchers working on a COVID-19 vaccine at the Vaccine Research Center at the National Institute of Allergy and Infectious Diseases; Kathrin Jansen, the Head of Vaccine Research and Development for Pfizer, is another towering vaccine leader.

Apart from scientists, there are many women leaders who have ensured distribution and administration of COVID-19 vaccines. Dr Soumya Swaminathan, the WHO's Chief Scientist; Dr Ngozi Ikonji-Iweala, the Chair of the GAVI Alliance, and Jane Halton, the Chair of the Coalition for Epidemic Preparedness, have played key roles in the development of the COVAX initiative. Aurélia Nguyen, the Managing Director of the COVAX facility, has brought 186 countries together. Anuradha Gupta, Deputy CEO of GAVI, has played a key role in equitable distribution of vaccines. Mariangela Simao, the Assistant Director General of the WHO for Drug Access, Vaccines and Pharmaceuticals Division, and Professor Kate O'Brien, the Director of Vaccines and Biologics at the WHO, are other key leaders.

GRASSROOT LEADERSHIP: BRAVING BULLETS AND BOMBS

Leadership is essential in successful mass vaccination campaigns, not only at the political or scientific level, but also at the frontline. Leaders at the grassroots include doctors, nurses, community health workers and volunteers. They are trusted sources of information and bearers of messages about the benefits and safety of vaccines.[71,72]

Once unthinkable, the feat of smallpox eradication could be achieved because of the strong backbone of millions of ground leaders who spearheaded the vaccination drive under incredible circumstances.[73] Similarly, in eradication of polio, the frontline leaders were instrumental in rallying community support for vaccination.[74] Grassroot leaders walked miles, in rain and scorching heat, knee-deep snow and even in neck-deep water to administer polio drops.[75] Innumerable workers succumbed to bullets and bombs during immunization campaigns.[76,77] Many more suffered beating, abuses and aggressive resistance.[78]

In the COVID-19 campaign as well, the health workers and volunteers at the frontlines worked tirelessly to overcome entrenched vaccination hesitancy and reach eligible people. They used innovative ways to make mass vaccination a success.

When India crossed the formidable mark of one billion vaccinations, the Prime Minister Modi rightly dedicated the success of India's vaccination drive to its frontline vaccine leaders.[79]

TRADITIONAL AND RELIGIOUS LEADERS

Another class of leaders who have the potential to change the face of any mass vaccination campaign are the traditional and religious leaders. They have been associated with inoculations from the pre-vaccine era. The first written account of variolation describes a Buddhist nun powdering scabs taken from a smallpox patient and blowing them into a healthy person to induce immunity.[81]

People trust religious leaders, give credence to their words and look to them for guidance. This gives them enormous 'social capital, which should be harnessed to dispel rumours, eliminate myths and spread positive messages about vaccination.

Many countries have relied on religious leaders to make mass vaccination drives successful. They have imparted training to these leaders to enhance their knowledge of vaccination and sharpen their leadership skills.[82,83]

In India, religious leaders have played a positive role in mobilizing strong support for vaccination. They helped to eliminate myths and misconceptions about vaccines and softened resistance in underserved areas.[84] Religious leaders have played a key role in eradication of smallpox and polio from India. They have been roped in to promote other vaccines as well. For example, in November 2018, the Chief Minister of Uttar Pradesh, Yogi Adityanath, who is a religious leader, launched a campaign (with religious leaders) to promote the measles and rubella vaccines. Sunni leader Maulana Khalid Rasheed Firangi Mahli; Maulana Arshad Madni, President of the Jamait-e-ulama-hind Deoband; Chief of the Mankameshwar Temple, Mahant Devya Giri, and Rev. Father George D'Costa joined the campaign.[85]

Initially, clerics in Nigeria rejected the polio vaccine, causing setbacks to the polio eradication initiative. The tide turned starting in 2003 with the active engagement of traditional and religious leaders.[86] The Majigi, a community communication and awareness campaign, was launched in 2008 to systematically engage Muslims and Christian clerics to promote acceptance of polio vaccination.[87,88]

In the case of COVID-19, people have reported a high degree of trust in the clergy.[89] The Vatican and the US Conference of Catholic Bishops have called vaccination 'an act of charity toward the other members of our community'.[90] Pope Francis said that being vaccinated is everyone's moral obligation, since it helps to preserve not only the individual's life, but also that of others.[91]

In India too, religious leaders have played a critical role in exploding myths and promoting COVID-19 vaccination. The Federal Ministry of Minority Affairs launched a pan-India campaign, 'Jaan Hai To Jahan Hai' (If you have life, you have the world) to tackle concerns and myths about the COVID-19 vaccine. A large number of leaders of different religions participated in the campaign. They included Syed Ahmed Bukhari, the Shahi Imam of Delhi's Jama Masjid; Jain religious leader Acharya Lokesh Muni; Manjinder Singh Sirsa, President of the Delhi Sikh Gurdwara Management Committee, and Dr Umer Ahmed Ilyasi, Chief Imam of the All India Imam Organization.[92]

ORGANIZATIONAL LEADERS

Mass vaccination campaigns require mobilization of experts, civil society and volunteers as well as sharing of scientific and medical breakthroughs. The spectrum of vaccination leadership is not complete without organizational leaders who facilitate these tasks.

WHO: The Global Institutional Leader

The WHO, established in 1948, is the global institution that is mandated to deal with pandemics. It is the coordinating and directing authority on international health within the UN. The WHO has spearheaded the eradication of smallpox and polio campaigns.

In the case of smallpox, the WHO assumed global leadership for its eradication in 1959. It launched the Intensified Smallpox Eradication Program, which included two main components: detection, monitoring and investigation of smallpox cases and mass vaccination.

Smallpox was eradicated in 1980, marking the end of a disease that had plagued humanity for at least 3,000 years, killing

300 million people in the 20th century alone. Smallpox eradication-related efforts and learning led to the launch of the Expanded Program of Immunization by the WHO in 1974 for tuberculosis, DPT, measles, polio, hepatitis B and yellow fever.[21] In 1988, the WHO launched its Global Polio Eradication Initiative (GPEI) to eradicate the disease by 2000.

In May 2012, the WHO adopted the Global Vaccine Action Plan (GVAP) to prevent millions of deaths by 2020 through equitable access to existing vaccines for people in all communities.[93]

The COVID-19 pandemic was a moment of reckoning for the WHO, which launched numerous initiatives to mass vaccinate people. These initiatives include the ACT Accelerator and the COVAX facility. As I write, 172 countries are participating in COVAX and over 1.43 billion COVID-19 vaccines have been delivered to 145 countries.[94] The WHO has also launched a solidarity vaccine trial to evaluate the safety, efficiency, reliability and efficacy of COVID-19 vaccine candidates.

The WHO has sensitized world leaders about the critical importance of quick availability and administration of effective vaccines against COVID-19. It has also made repeated requests to redistribute, fund and increase the availability of vaccines.[95]

GAVI: The Vaccine Alliance

GAVI, the vaccine alliance, was created in 2000 by the WHO, the UNICEF, the World Bank and the Bill & Melinda Gates Foundation. GAVI's mission is to save children's lives and protect their health by promoting equitable and sustainable use of vaccines and strengthening health systems to deliver immunization services.[96]

GAVI works with manufacturers to ensure that vaccines are available at affordable rates. In return, it offers long-term, high-volume and predictable demand. Because of its market-shaping efforts, the cost of total immunization of a child with all

11 WHO-recommended childhood vaccines costs $28 in Gavi-supported countries, compared to $1,200 in the USA.[97]

GAVI now helps to vaccinate almost half the world's children against deadly and debilitating infectious diseases. It also supports delivery and introduction of new and lifesaving vaccines to the world's poorest countries.[98] During the COVID-19 pandemic, GAVI was at the centre of the international response. It coordinated COVAX with the CEPI, the WHO and UNICEF.

Coalition for Epidemic Preparedness Innovations

The CEPI was launched in 2017 in the aftermath of the Ebola outbreak in West Africa. It is a global partnership between private, public, philanthropic and civil organizations. Its partners include the governments of Norway, India, Japan, the United Kingdom, the European Union, the Bill & Melinda Gates Foundation, the Welcome Trust and the World Economic Forum.

The CEPI aims to develop new ways of stimulating, co-ordinating and financing accelerated development of safe, effective and affordable vaccines in adequate quantity and in time for new pathogens.

Since its launch in 2017, the CEPI has mobilized more than $750 million to support its mission. Before COVID-19, it focused on developing vaccines against the Ebola virus, the Lassa virus, the MERS coronavirus, the Nipah virus, the Rift Valley Fever virus and the Chikungunya virus. The CEPI has also invested in new platform technologies to accelerate the response time to unexpected epidemic threats.[99,100]

On 10 March 2021, the CEPI launched an ambitious five-year $3.5 billion roadmap to compress vaccine development timelines to 100 days, develop a broadly protective vaccine against COVID-19, address new priorities and create a 'library' of vaccine candidates for use against known and unknown pathogens.[101]

Bill and Melinda Gates Foundation

The Bill & Melinda Gates Foundation was established by Bill Gates and his wife, Melinda Gates, in 2000. The foundation works in more than 100 countries. Its objectives include a reduction in morbidity and mortality from vaccine-preventable diseases. To achieve this, it supports increased access to existing vaccines and research into affordable and effective new vaccines.[103,104]

The Gates Foundation, as it is commonly called, is the founding partner of GAVI, the vaccine alliance. Through GAVI, the Foundation has been able to focus international attention on the need for mass immunization. The Foundation has also announced Bill and Melinda Gates' Children's Vaccine Program with a financial commitment of $750 million. The programme's aim is to accelerate access to new vaccines for children living in poor countries.[105]

To ensure that the world sees the back of the COVID-19 pandemic, the Foundation has contributed liberally to the COVAX AMC of the GAVI. It also supported the development of the Indian vaccine COVISHIELD.[106]

The Foundation has announced a $20 million grant to the CEPI. This donation is aimed at advancing research and jumpstarting the development of promising vaccine candidates.[107]

Rotary International

Rotary International is known for its leadership in mass administration of polio vaccination globally. Rotary's fight against polio began on 29 September 1979 when it kick-started the Philippine poliomyelitis immunization campaign, which was aimed at immunizing around six million children.[108]

In 1981, Rotary decided to immunize children the world over against polio by 2005. In 1985, Rotary International launched its immunization programme, 'Polio Plus'.[109] When, in 1988, the WHO launched its GPEI, Rotary International became its international partner.[110] Millions of Rotary members volunteered their time and resources for the cause.[111,112]

Rotary also made an important contribution in the fight against COVID-19. The president of the organization appealed to its members globally to use their polio eradication experience, raise awareness about the importance of vaccination in their communities and support health workers in their vaccination efforts.

United Nations International Children's Emergency Fund

The United Nations International Children's Emergency Fund (UNICEF) is another global mass immunization leader. It came into being in 1946 and now works in 190 countries and territories.[113]

Since 1974, UNICEF has supported the delivery of immunization services globally. It has become the world's single-largest vaccine buyer and procures more than two billion vaccines annually. This helps it shape markets, cut costs and increase efficiency. UNICEF claims to have reached more than 760 million children with vaccines in the last two decades.[114]

UNICEF also works on maintenance and improvement of vaccine cold chains and strengthening of the front-line immunization workforce. It is also an active partner of the GPEI and manages procurement and distribution of more than one billion OPV doses. UNICEF also works with governments in developing action plans, eradication policies, training materials, advocacy, resource mobilization and logistics.[115]

UNICEF has facilitated vaccination in conflict-affected regions by negotiating peace corridors and days of tranquillity with the warring factions to allow access to vaccinators. It played a key role in vaccinating people against COVID-19 through the COVAX facility. It has used its market shaping and procurement-related expertise and existing infrastructure to coordinate procurement and supply of COVID-19 vaccines for COVAX. UNICEF also procures and supplies immunization necessities such as syringes, safety boxes for their disposal and CCE such as vaccine refrigerators.[116]

The vaccine journey has been incredible. Many towering milestones have been reached through sheer hard work, innovation, sacrifices and entrepreneurship. Let us take a look at the future prospects and challenges of the miracle known as 'vaccine'.

REFERENCES

1. OECD. 2021. Enhancing public trust in COVID-19 vaccination: The role of governments [online]. Available from: https://www.oecd.org/coronavirus/policy-responses/enhancing-public-trust-in-covid-19-vaccination-the-role-of-governments-eae0ec5a/
2. Crosby BC, Bryson JM. *Leadership for the common good: Tackling public problems in a shared-power world.* Hoboken, NJ: John Wiley & Sons; 2005.
3. Saleh, J., 2015. Public health leadership theory in immunization campaigns: A look at the transactional and transformational leaderships styles [online]. Available from: <https://www.researchgate.net/publication/280580041_Public_Health_Leadership_Theory_In_Immunization_Campaigns_a_look_at_the_Transactional_and_Transformational_Leaderships_Styles
4. Durch JS. Overcoming barriers to immunization: A workshop summary.
5. Osborn RN, Hunt JG, Jauch LR. Toward a contextual theory of leadership. *The Leadership Quarterly*. 2002 December;13(6):797–837.
6. Emperor Of China Kangxi [online]. Encyclopedia.com. 2020. Available from: https://www.encyclopedia.com/people/history/chinese-and-taiwanese-history-biographies/emperor-china-kangxi
7. Weiss R A, J Esparza. The prevention and eradication of smallpox: a commentary on Sloane (1755) 'An account of inoculation'. *Philosophical Transactions of the Royal Society B: Biological Sciences*. 2015 April; 370(1666):20140378.
8. Hajj HI, Chams N, Chams S, Sayegh S El, Badran R, Raad M, Gerges-Geagea A, Leone A, Urjus JA. Vaccines through centuries: Major cornerstones of global health. *Frontiers in Public Health*. 2015 November 26;3:269.
9. Historic UK. 2021. Lady Mary Wortley Montagu and her campaign against smallpox—historic UK [online]. Available from: https://www.historic-uk.com/HistoryUK/HistoryofBritain/Lady-Mary-Wortley-Montagu-Campaign-Against-Smallpox/

10. Who was Lady Mary Wortley Montagu? [Internet]. National Trust. 2021 [cited 10 December 2021]. Available from: https://www.nationaltrust.org.uk/features/who-was-lady-mary-wortley-montagu
11. Chichowlas O. Catherine the Great Smallpox Letter Echoes Russia's Pandemic Woes [Internet]. *The Moscow Times*. 2021 [cited 10 December 2021]. Available from: https://www.themoscowtimes.com/2021/11/19/catherine-the-great-smallpox-letter-echoes-russias-pandemic-woes-a75614
12. Timeline. History of vaccines [Internet]. Historyofvaccines.org. 2021 [cited 10 December 2021]. Available from: https://www.historyofvaccines.org/timeline#EVT_43
13. Troops G. Gen. George Washington ordered smallpox inoculations for all troops [Internet]. Military Health System. 2021 [cited 10 December 2021]. Available from: https://health.mil/News/Articles/2021/08/16/Gen-George-Washington-Ordered-Smallpox-Inoculations-for-All-Troops
14. Statesman.com. 2021 [cited 10 December 2021]. Available from: https://www.statesman.com/story/news/politics/politifact/2021/08/02/did-george-washington-mandate-vaccines-smallpox-continental-army-during-revolutionary-war/5456106001/
15. Werther R. George Washington and the first mandatory immunization. *Journal of the American Revolution* [Internet]. *Journal of the American Revolution*. 2021 [cited 10 December 2021]. Available from: https://allthingsliberty.com/2021/10/george-washington-and-the-first-mandatory-immunization/
16. The right to health [Internet]. Nytimes.com. 2021 [cited 10 December 2021]. Available from: https://www.nytimes.com/2021/09/30/briefing/vaccine-mandate-covid.html
17. Youngdahl K. American presidents and infectious diseases. History of Vaccines [Internet]. Historyofvaccines.org. 2013 [cited 10 December 2021]. Available from: https://www.historyofvaccines.org/content/blog/american-presidents-and-infectious-diseases
18. Inoculation. Thomas Jefferson's Monticello [Internet]. Monticello.org. 2021 [cited 10 December 2021]. Available from: https://www.monticello.org/site/research-and-collections/inoculation
19. Rigau-Pérez JG. The real philanthropic expedition of the smallpox vaccine: monarchy and modernity in 1803. *Puerto Rico Health Sciences Journal*. 2004 September 1;23(3):223–231.
20. Botet FA. Fighting against smallpox around the world. The vaccination expeditions of Xavier de Balmis (1803–1806) and Josep Salvany (1803–1810). *Contributions to Science*. 2012 October 31;99–105.
21. Andrus JK, Bandyopadhyay AS, Danovaro-Holliday M, Dietz V, Domingues C, Figueroa JP, et al. The past, present, and future of immunization in the Americas. *RevistaPanamericana de SaludPública*. 2018 April 12;41:e121.

22. Tarrago R. The Balmis-Salvany smallpox expedition: the first public health vaccination campaign in South America. *Perspectives in Health (PAHO)*. 2001;6(1).
23. Origin of our name [Internet]. Marchofdimes.org. 2021 [cited 10 December 2021]. Available from: https://www.marchofdimes.org/mission/eddie-cantor-and-the-origin-of-the-march-of-dimes.aspx
24. Berish A. FDR and polio. FDR Presidential Library and Museum [Internet]. Fdrlibrary.org. 2021 [cited 10 December 2021]. Available from: https://www.fdrlibrary.org/polio
25. Gelfand HM. A critical examination of the Indian smallpox eradication program. *American Journal of Public Health and the Nations Health*. 1966 October;56(10):1634–1651.
26. Ghosh S. How India nixed smallpox [Internet]. 2021 [cited 10 December 2021]. Available from: https://thepatriot.in/2020/03/27/how-india-ixed-smallpox/
27. Ogden HG. CDC and the Smallpox Crusade. US Department of Health and Human Services, Public Health Service, Centers for Disease Control. 1987.
28. Chatterjee K. India's war on smallpox: Lessons for the Covid19 pandemic. Live History India [Internet]. Live History India. 2021 [cited 10 December 2021]. Available from: https://www.livehistoryindia.com/story/mmi-cover-story/smallpox/
29. Fenner F, Henderson DA, Arita I, Jezek Z, Ladnyi ID. Smallpox and its eradication. Geneva: World Health Organization. 2 March 1988.
30. Samnani AA. Political economy of poliomyelitis (India case study). Available from: https://internalmedicine.imedpub.com/political-economy-of-poliomyelitis-india-case-study.php?aid=9902
31. GPEI. How India eradicated polio [Internet]. Polioeradication.org. 2021 [cited 10 December 2021]. Available from: https://polioeradication.org/news-post/how-india-eradicated-polio-challenges-and-lessons-learned/
32. India: A push to vaccinate every child, everywhere ended polio in India [Internet]. Who.int. 2021 [cited 10 December 2021]. Available from: https://www.who.int/india/news/feature-stories/detail/a-push-to-vaccinate-every-child-everywhere-ended-polio-in-india
33. Polio eradication efforts in India. 2021 [cited 10 December 2021]. Available from: https://main.mohfw.gov.in/sites/default/files/Pulse%20Polio%20Programme.pdf
34. PM Modi's visit to vaccine facilities acknowledgement of institutions built over decades: Anand Sharma [Internet]. *Deccan Herald*. 2021 [cited 10 December 2021]. Available from: https://www.deccanherald.com/national/national-politics/pm-modis-visit-to-vaccine-facilities-acknowledgement-of-institutions-built-over-decades-anand-sharma-921365.html
35. Modi meets COVID-19 vaccine manufacturers [Internet]. *The Hindu*. 2021 [cited 10 December 2021]. Available from: https://www.thehindu.

com/news/national/pm-modi-meets-indian-covid-vaccine-manufacturers/article37139056.ece
36. Ramesh P. Modi's pandemic leadership [Internet]. *Open the Magazine.* 2021 [cited 10 December 2021]. Available from: https://openthemagazine.com/cover-stories/modis-pandemic-leadership/
37. Express Web Desk. PM Modi flags complacency, asks officials to take Covid vaccination drive door to door [Internet]. *The Indian Express.* 2021 [cited 10 December 2021]. Available from: https://indianexpress.com/article/india/narendra-modi-covid-vaccination-districts-door-to-door-create-awareness-misconceptions-7605688/
38. Narendra Modi calls for door-to-door COVID-19 vaccination [Internet]. *The Hindu.* 2021 [cited 10 December 2021]. Available from: https://www.thehindu.com/news/national/pm-holds-review-meeting-with-dms-of-over-40-districts-on-low-covid-vaccination-coverage/article37317930.ece
39. The fight over inoculation during the 1721 Boston smallpox epidemic [Internet]. *Science in the News.* 2021 [cited 10 December 2021]. Available from: https://sitn.hms.harvard.edu/flash/special-edition-on-infectious-disease/2014/the-fight-over-inoculation-during-the-1721-boston-smallpox-epidemic/
40. Hoffman D. The man who defeated smallpox [Internet]. Foreign Policy. 2021 [cited 10 December 2021]. Available from: https://foreignpolicy.com/2010/05/05/the-man-who-defeated-smallpox/
41. Donald A. Henderson. Johns Hopkins Bloomberg School of Public Health [Internet]. Johns Hopkins Bloomberg School of Public Health. 2021 [cited 10 December 2021]. Available from: https://publichealth.jhu.edu/about/history/heroes-of-public-health/donald-a-henderson
42. Dr Donald A. Henderson. PAHO/WHO. Pan American Health Organization [Internet]. Paho.org. 2021 [cited 10 December 2021]. Available from: https://www.paho.org/en/public-health-heroes/dr-donald-henderson
43. Access to COVID-19 Tools (ACT) Accelerator [Internet]. WHO.int. 2021 [cited 10 December 2021]. Available from: https://www.who.int/initiatives/act-accelerator
44. WHO chief says unfair COVID-19 vaccine distribution risks causing 'catastrophic moral failure'. World News. *Firstpost* [Internet]. *Firstpost.* 2021 [cited 10 December 2021]. Available from: https://www.firstpost.com/world/who-chief-says-unfair-covid-19-vaccine-distribution-risks-causing-catastrophic-moral-failure-9215801.html
45. WHO chief Tedros Adhanom Ghebreyesus unbowed amid attacks Trump criticism [Internet]. *The Economic Times.* 2021 [cited 10 December 2021]. Available from: https://economictimes.indiatimes.com/news/international/world-news/un-health-agency-chief-unbowed-amid-attacks-trump-criticism/articleshow/75734049.cms?utm_source=contentofinterest&utm_medium=text&utm_campaign=cppst

46. Baxby D. The Jenner bicentenary: the introduction and early distribution of smallpox vaccine. *FEMS Immunology & Medical Microbiology*. 1996 November 1;16(1):1–10.
47. Behbehani AM. The smallpox story: life and death of an old disease. *Microbiological Review*. 1983 December;47(4):455–509.
48. About Edward Jenner—The Jenner Institute [Internet]. 2021 [cited 10 December 2021]. Available from: https://www.jenner.ac.uk/about/edward-jenner
49. Waterhouse Benjamin. To slay the devouring monster. OnView. Digital Collections & Exhibits [Internet]. Collections.countway.harvard.edu. 2021 [cited 10 December 2021]. Available from: https://collections.countway.harvard.edu/onview/exhibits/show/to-slay-the-devouring-monster/benjamin-waterhouse
50. The College of Physicians of Philadelphia. *History of Vaccines Timelines*. The College of Physicians of Philadelphia; 1885. Available from: https://collegeofphysicians.org/our-work/history-vaccines
51. Smallpox vaccination and the waterhouse experiments. Gilt by Association. *OnView*: Digital Collections & Exhibits [Internet]. Collections.countway.harvard.edu. 2021 [cited 10 December 2021]. Available from: https://collections.countway.harvard.edu/onview/exhibits/show/gilt/smallpox
52. Esparza J, Lederman S, Nitsche A, Damaso CR. Early smallpox vaccine manufacturing in the United States: introduction of the animal vaccine in 1870; establishment of 'vaccine farms' and the beginnings of the vaccine industry. *Vaccine*. 2020 June 19;38(30):4773–4779.
53. Hansen B. Smallpox and the long road to eradication [Internet]. Science History Institute. 2021 [cited 10 December 2021]. Available from: https://www.sciencehistory.org/distillations/smallpox-and-the-long-road-to-eradication
54. Prabhu M. The age of modern vaccines: An abridged history of vaccines, Part 2 [Internet]. GAVI.org. 2021 [cited 10 December 2021]. Available from: https://www.gavi.org/vaccineswork/age-modern-vaccines-abridged-history-vaccines-part-2
55. Smith K A. Louis Pasteur: The father of immunology? *Frontiers in Immunology*. 10 April 2012. 3:68.
56. Mehta P. Adopt an offensive strategy for key economic decisions [Internet]. *Mint*. 2021 [cited 10 December 2021]. Available from: https://www.livemint.com/opinion/online-views/adopt-an-offensive-strategy-for-key-economic-decisions-11608825978628.html
57. Hawgood BJ. Waldemar Mordecai Haffkine, CIE (1860–1930): Prophylactic vaccination against cholera and bubonic plague in British India. *Journal of Medical Biography*. 2007 February;15(1):9–19.
58. Sorokina M. Between faith and reason. Waldemar Haffkine (1860–1930) in India. In: Robbins WX, Tokayer M, editors. *Western Jews in India: From the Fifteenth Century to the Present*. New Delhi: Manohar Publishers; 2013. 161–178.

59. The last resort: The man who saved the world from two pandemics [Internet]. The Librarians. 2021 [cited 10 December 2021]. Available from: https://blog.nli.org.il/en/haffkine/
60. Chen I, Humeniuk H. Outstanding scientist and bacteriologist Waldemar Haffkine [Internet]. 2021 [cited 10 December 2021]. Available from: https://www.researchgate.net/publication/346480482_Outstanding_scientist_and_bacteriologist_Waldemar_Haffkine
61. Gunter J, Pandey V. Waldemar Haffkine: The vaccine pioneer the world forgot [Internet]. *BBC News*. 2021 [cited 10 December 2021]. Available from: https://www.bbc.com/news/world-asia-india-55050012
62. Jishnu L. Wishing for a Jonas Salk in the age of COVID-19 [Internet]. Downtoearth.org.in. 2021 [cited 10 December 2021]. Available from: https://www.downtoearth.org.in/blog/health/wishing-for-a-jonas-salk-in-the-age-of-covid-19-74822
63. About Jonas Salk [Internet]. Salk Institute for Biological Studies. 2021 [cited 10 December 2021]. Available from: https://www.salk.edu/about/history-of-salk/jonas-salk/
64. Tan SY, Ponstein N. Jonas Salk (1914–1995): A vaccine against polio. *Singapore Medical Journal*. 2019 January;60(1):9
65. Salk Jonas, Albert Bruce Sabin [Internet]. Science History Institute. 2021 [cited 10 December 2021]. Available from: https://www.sciencehistory.org/historical-profile/jonas-salk-and-albert-bruce-sabin
66. Saxena A. World polio day: A look at India's journey towards becoming polio-free nation [Internet]. Thelogicalindian.com. 2021 [cited 10 December 2021]. Available from: https://thelogicalindian.com/health/world-polio-day-india-31442
67. The first century of women in vaccine science: 1970s to 1990s (Part 3). *Absolutely Maybe* [Internet]. *Absolutely Maybe*. 2022 [cited 19 January 2022]. Available from: https://absolutelymaybe.plos.org/2021/08/31/the-first-century-of-women-in-vaccine-science-1970s-1990s-part-3/
68. The vital and overlooked women who pioneered vaccines throughout history [Internet]. inews.co.uk. 2022 [cited 19 January 2022]. Available from: https://inews.co.uk/opinion/international-womens-day-2021-women-pioneered-vaccines-history-892545
69. Pioneering work of women scientists in India gets a boost [Internet]. IndBiz. Economic Diplomacy Division. 2022 [cited 19 January 2022]. Available from: https://indbiz.gov.in/pioneering-work-of-women-scientists-in-india-gets-a-boost/
70. Bora S. Meet 10 female scientists instrumental in developing COVID-19 vaccines around the world [Internet]. SheThePeople TV. 2021 [cited 10 December 2021]. Available from: https://www.shethepeople.tv/home-top-video/meet-10-female-scientists-instrumental-in-developing-covid-19-v;accines-around-the-world/

71. Rosen BL, Goodson P, Thompson B, Wilson KL. School nurses' knowledge, attitudes, perceptions of role as opinion leader, and professional practice regarding human papillomavirus vaccine for youth. *Journal of School Health*. 2015 February;85(2):73–81.
72. Pauvrete V. How frontline health workers are writing India's immunization success story [Internet]. *Global Citizen*. 2021 [cited 10 December 2021]. Available from: https://www.globalcitizen.org/fr/content/frontline-health-workers-immunization-success/
73. Roychowdhury A. In India's eradication of smallpox and polio, lessons on how to (and how not to) tackle Covid-19 vaccination [Internet]. *The Indian Express*. 2021 [cited 10 December 2021]. Available from: https://indianexpress.com/article/research/in-indias-eradication-of-smallpox-and-polio-lesson-on-how-to-and-how-not-to-tackle-covid-19-vaccination-7310266/
74. India's health workers: Ending polio is just the beginning [Internet]. *Global Citizen*. 2021 [cited 10 December 2021]. Available from: https://www.globalcitizen.org/en/content/indias-health-workers-ending-polio-is-just-the-beg/
75. GPEI. The linchpin of on-ground polio eradication: women health workers and leaders [Internet]. Polioeradication.org. 2021 [cited 10 December 2021]. Available from: https://polioeradication.org/news-post/the-linchpin-of-on-ground-polio-eradication-women-health-workers-and-leaders/
76. IED blast injures lady health worker (2013). *The Express Tribune*. Available from: http://tribune.com.pk/story/516158/ied-blast-injures-lady-health-worker/
77. Tank killing: Lady health worker shot dead (2013). *The Express Tribune*. Available from: http://tribune.com.pk/story/572624/tank-killing-lady-health-worker-shot-dead/
78. Closser S, Jooma R. Why we must provide better support for Pakistan's female frontline health workers. PLoS medicine. 2013 October;10(10): e1001528.
79. PM praises frontline, health workers as India administers over 2 crore doses [Internet]. NDTV.com. 2021 [cited 10 December 2021]. Available from: https://www.ndtv.com/india-news/pm-praises-frontline-health-workers-as-india-administers-over-2-crore-doses-2544891
80. Zarocostas J. UNICEF taps religious leaders in vaccination push. *The Lancet*. 2004 May 22;363(9422):1709.
81. Grabenstein JD. What the world's religions teach, applied to vaccines and immune globulins. *Vaccine*. 2013;31(16):2011–2023.
82. UNICEF. Building trust in immunization: Partnering with religious leaders and groups. New York, NY: UNICEF; 2004. 23–26.
83. Oyo-Ita A, Bosch-Capblanch X, Ross A, Oku A, Esu E, Ameh S, et al. Effects of engaging communities in decision-making and action through traditional and religious leaders on vaccination coverage in Cross River

State, Nigeria: A cluster-randomised control trial. *Plos One*. 2021 April 16;16(4):e0248236.

84. India is polio-free: What can Pakistan, Afghanistan and Nigeria learn? [Internet]. *The Guardian*. 2021 [cited 10 December 2021]. Available from: https://www.theguardian.com/global-development-professionals-network/2014/jan/13/lessons-india-polio-free-landmark
85. Religious leaders advocate measles-rubella campaign [Internet]. *Times of India*. 2018 [cited 19 January 2022]. Available from: https://timesofindia.indiatimes.com/city/lucknow/religious-leaders-advocate-for-measles-rubella-campaign/articleshow/66822506.cms
86. Thissen P, Rao K. Evidence impact: Increasing immunization rates by engaging community leaders [Internet]. 3ieimpact.org. 2021 [cited 10 December 2021]. Available from: https://www.3ieimpact.org/blogs/evidence-impact-increasing-immunization-rates-engaging-community-leaders
87. Mohammed A, Tomori O, Nkengasong JN. Lessons from elimination of poliomyelitis in Africa. *Nature Reviews Immunology*. 2021 December;21(12):823–828.
88. Nasir SG, Aliyu G, Ya'u I, Gadanya M, Mohammad M, Zubair M, El-Kamary SS. From intense rejection to advocacy: How Muslim clerics were engaged in a polio eradication initiative in Northern Nigeria. *PLoS Medicine*. 2014 August 5;11(8):e1001687.
89. Nortey J, Lipika M. Most Americans would trust their clergy's COVID-19 vaccine advice [Internet]. Pew Research Center's Religion & Public Life Project. 2021 [cited 10 December 2021]. Available from: https://www.pewforum.org/2021/10/15/most-americans-who-go-to-religious-services-say-they-would-trust-their-clergys-advice-on-covid-19-vaccines/
90. Lehmann C. Faith leaders spread the word: Get vaccinated [Internet]. WebMD. 2021 [cited 10 December 2021]. Available from: https://www.webmd.com/vaccines/covid-19-vaccine/news/20210126/faith-leaders-spread-the-word-get-vaccinated
91. Galang JR. Science and religion for COVID-19 vaccine promotion. *Journal of Public Health*. 2021 September 22;43(3):e513–e514.
92. 'Jaan Hai To Jahan Hai' Covid vaccine awareness campaign to start From 21 June [Internet]. NDTV.com. 2021 [cited 19 January 2022]. Available from: https://www.ndtv.com/india-news/minority-affairs-ministry-to-launch-jaan-hai-to-jahan-hai-covid-19-vaccine-awareness-campaign-on-june-21-2467617
93. Global vaccine action plan [Internet]. WHO.int. 2021 [cited 10 December 2021]. Available from: https://www.who.int/teams/immunization-vaccines-and-biologicals/strategies/global-vaccine-action-plan
94. Covax. 1 billion doses delivered [Internet]. GAVI.org. 2022 [cited 19 January 2022]. Available from: https://www.gavi.org/covax-vaccine-roll-out

95. Laskar R. WHO-appointed panel slams slow response to Covid-19 in 2020, seeks more powers for UN body [Internet]. *Hindustan Times*. 2021 [cited 10 December 2021]. Available from: https://www.hindustantimes.com/world-news/who-appointed-panel-slams-slow-response-to-covid-19-in-2020-seeks-more-powers-for-un-body-101620839204846.html
96. WHO-GAVI. The global alliance for vaccines and immunizations [Internet]. WHO.int. 2021 [cited 10 December 2021]. Available from: https://www.who.int/workforcealliance/members_partners/member_list/gavi/en/
97. Lob-Levyt J. Special event on philanthropy and the global public health agenda [Internet]. Un.org. 2021 [cited 10 December 2021]. Available from: https://www.un.org/en/ecosoc/phlntrpy/docs/gavi.pdf
98. GAVI at 20: How far have we come and how far can we go? [Internet]. Results UK. 2021 [cited 10 December 2021]. Available from: https://www.results.org.uk/blog/gavi-20-how-far-have-we-come-and-how-far-can-we-go
99. Why we exist? CEPI [Internet]. CEPI. 2021 [cited 10 December 2021]. Available from: https://cepi.net/about/whyweexist/
100. WHO.int. 2021 [cited 10 December 2021]. Available from: https://www.who.int/immunization/sage/meetings/2019/april/1_CEPI_Summary_WHO_SAGE_Meeting_April.pdf
101. Samarasekera U. CEPI prepares for future pandemics and epidemics. *The Lancet* Infectious Diseases. 2021 May1;21(5):608.
102. Bill and Melinda Gates Foundation: What is it and what does it do? [Internet]. *BBC News*. 2021 [cited 10 December 2021]. Available from: https://www.bbc.com/news/world-us-canada-56979480
103. Gates Foundation. American organization [Internet]. Encyclopedia Britannica. 2021 [cited 10 December 2021]. Available from: https://www.britannica.com/topic/Gates-Foundation
104. Bill & Melinda Gates Foundation [Internet]. Oecd-ilibrary.org. 2021 [cited 10 December 2021]. Available from: https://www.oecd-ilibrary.org/sites/da5658fd-en/index.html?itemId=/content/component/da5658fd-en
105. Bill and Melinda Gates call for collaboration innovation to deliver COVID 19 breakthroughs [Internet]. Bill and Melinda Gates Foundation. 2021 [cited 10 December 2021]. Available from: https://www.gatesfoundation.org/ideas/media-center/press-releases/2020/12/bill-and-melinda-gates-call-for-collaboration-innovation-to-deliver-covid-19-breakthroughs
106. Bill Gates: The virus and the quest to vaccinate the world (Published 2020) [Internet]. Nytimes.com. 2021 [cited 10 December 2021]. Available from: https://www.nytimes.com/2020/11/23/world/bill-gates-vaccine-coronavirus.html
107. Gates Foundation announces new funds to develop COVID-19 vaccines and increase access to affordable vaccines in low-income countries [Internet]. Bill and Melinda Gates Foundation. 2021 [cited 10 December 2021]. Available from: https://www.gatesfoundation.org/ideas/media-center/

press-releases/2020/11/gates-foundation-announces-new-funds-to-develop-covid-19-vaccines

108. Rotary polio eradication efforts [Internet]. Rotary.org. 2021 [cited 10 December 2021]. Available from: https://www.rotary.org/en/history-rotary-polio-eradication-efforts

109. Bhattacharya S, Dasgupta R. A tale or two global health programs. Smallpox eradication's lessons for the Antipolio campaign in India. American *Journal of Public Health*. 2009 July;99(7):1176–1184.

110. Vaccines to end polio: Rotary lead the way [Internet]. GAVI.org. 2021 [cited 10 December 2021]. Available from: https://www.gavi.org/vaccines-to-end-polio-rotary-lead-the-way

111. GPEI Partners [Internet]. Polioeradication.org. 2021 [cited 10 December 2021]. Available from: https://polioeradication.org/who-we-are/partners/

112. Dochterman C. Rotary's involvement in polio eradication [Internet]. Clubrunner.blob.core.windows.net. 2021 [cited 10 December 2021]. Available from: https://clubrunner.blob.core.windows.net/00000001415/en-ca/files/homepage/rotary-s-invovlement-in-polio-eradication/Rotarys-involvement-in-Polio-Eradication.pdf

113. Through pandemics and epidemics, hope stays alive [Internet]. Unicef.org. 2021 [cited 10 December 2021]. Available from: https://www.unicef.org/stories/through-pandemics-epidemics-hope-stays-alive

114. COVAX: Ensuring global equitable access to COVID-19 vaccines [Internet]. Unicef.org. 2021 [cited 10 December 2021]. Available from: https://www.unicef.org/supply/covax-ensuring-global-equitable-access-covid-19-vaccines

115. Albala S. Thematic analysis of the culture of UNICEF in response to polio eradication efforts. 2015. Available from: https://repository.upenn.edu/cgi/viewcontent.cgi?article=1000&context=anthro_seniortheses

116. Urgent action needed now to ensure sufficient COVID vaccine syringe supply to meet 2022 vaccination targets [Internet]. Unicef.org. 2021 [cited 10 December 2021]. Available from: https://www.unicef.org/press-releases/urgent-action-needed-now-ensure-sufficient-covid-vaccine-syringe-supply-meet-2022

Epilogue

New Arsenal, New Challenges

In their 225-year journey, vaccines have become the cornerstones of the management of infectious diseases. They have been pivotal in improving global health, saving millions of lives and enhancing human life expectancy.[1] Since Jenner's time, the world has witnessed a sea change in vaccine development and understanding of the immune system. However, the challenges posed by pathogens have multiplied as well.

THE PANDEMIC CENTURY

In the last 100 years, the world has braced itself against a series of epidemics and pandemics, including Ebola, Zika, the MERS pandemic, influenza, SARS and SARS-CoV-2.[2] More than 300 emerging infectious diseases have been identified.[3] At least seven coronaviruses, including SARS-CoV-2, have caused illnesses and deaths.[4,5]

The rate of animal-to-human spread of pathogens has gone up.[6,7] In zoonotic transmission, RNA viruses are posing a formidable public health concern. They have high mutation and recombination rates. Consequently, new viral strains emerge at a fast pace.[8]

VIRAL MUTATIONS: THE CHANGING FACES OF SARS-COV-2

The SARS-CoV-2 virus has mutated over time. The resultant genetic variation has implications for diagnostics and therapeutics,

including vaccination. SARS-CoV-2 mutations of concern included Alpha, Beta, Gamma, Delta and Omicron. Mutations of interest reported include Epsilon, Zeta, Eta, Theta, Iota and Kappa.

While Alpha was first noted in the United Kingdom in September 2020, Beta was first detected in South Africa in October 2020. The Delta variant was detected a couple of months thereafter and spread rapidly across the world, wreaking havoc. It was chiefly responsible for the second and deadlier wave of COVID-19 from May to June of 2021. This variant led to a second round of lockdown in many countries, including India. Delta is 60 per cent more transmissible than Alpha.

As life began to return to a new normal after Delta's wrath had subsided, the world faced another shock. It was the emergence of one more variant, called Omicron. While the variant spread fast, it was reported to be less deadly. Public health leaders and countries are watching, with their fingers crossed, the data on the efficacy of vaccines against this latest strain of the virus, the severity of the disease and the possibility of infection in people who have already recovered from COVID-19.

So are we losing ground to contagions that are evolving 40 million times faster?

IS THE WORLD LIKELY TO SEE MORE PANDEMICS?

Notwithstanding huge medical and scientific advancement, chances of epidemics and pandemics are constantly rising. Many bombs are ticking to erupt soon.[9] Increasing populations and the quest for development are not only bringing humans into increasing contact with each other, but also with animals that are reservoirs of novel pathogens.[10]

Apart from the sheer number, the proportion of older people who suffer from immunosenescence and consequently are vulnerable to a high risk of infection, has gone up.[11] An increase in cancer, obesity and resultant immunosuppression is also accelerating the transmission of diseases.[12,13,14]

Moreover, the global mobility of humans has increased tremendously. Annual air trips had gone up from 1 billion in 1990 to 4.2 billion in 2018.[15] Consequently, a contagion can spread from one corner of the world to another in hours.

People all over the world are migrating to cities. New urban spaces lack housing, sanitation and infrastructure. The people there live in overcrowded and unhygienic conditions, where contagion thrives. Climate change is also tilting the balance in favour of germs. Rising temperatures are increasing the range of animal and insect vectors humans are exposed to.[17] An increased risk of flooding, resulting from climate change, also increases the chances of outbreaks of waterborne diseases.

Wild animal markets and modern human-animal interactions are also multiplying the risk of disease outbreaks.[18] In addition, by use of genetic-engineering tools, terrorist groups or even a single person can unleash custom-designed virulent microbes.[2]

LESSONS IN VACCINOLOGY FROM COVID-19

COVID-19 turned out to be the severest pandemic of the century. Ultimately, it was the vaccine shield that rescued humanity from the onslaught of the SARS-CoV-2 virus. The brave fight against the contagion has taught numerous lessons on development and administration of vaccines.

COVID-19 validated novel technologies and quick ways of vaccine development. It ushered in an era of gene-based vaccine technologies, including DNA, mRNA and viral vector vaccines.[19] Before COVID-19, the development of a new vaccine would take about a decade. This was of little help in tackling disease outbreaks caused by novel pathogens. With new and nimbler platform technologies, scientists have successfully established a new paradigm for developing vaccines in less than 10 months.[20]

In COVID-19, vaccine makers learnt many lessons in vaccine development and operational excellence. These included simplified and innovative clinical trial designs and operations, the importance of taking sequential steps in parallel and combining phases of clinical trials. Predictive epidemiological modelling was used to identify emerging hot spots and select trial sites.[20]

COVID-19 also popularized the use of immunoinformatics, bioinformatics and AI in vaccine development.[1,21] There was real-time data-sharing, making critical information available quickly to the entire scientific community.[22] Chinese scientist, Zhang and his colleagues, sequenced the SARS-CoV-2 genome and made it publicly available as early as 10 January 2020.[23] This stimulated the work to identify antigenic epitopes. The first immunoinformatics-based SARS-CoV-2 vaccine construct was published in February 2020 and many more followed.[24]

The SARS-CoV-2 onslaught also taught us the benefits of a globally coordinated response for vaccine development.[19] The pandemic saw unprecedented cooperation between governments, private companies and academia. Global pharmaceutical and biotech companies, health authorities and regulatory agencies joined hands to defeat the pandemic. Their experience has made HICs realize although after the global economy lost trillions of dollars, that spending a few billions a year on research, surveillance, product development and manufacturing of vaccines in LMICs is beneficial for HICs.[20]

An important learning from COVID-19 is that adequate and timely financial support can work wonders in development of new vaccines. Governments and companies have invested billions of dollars, and that too is at risk, even before the vaccines were approved.[25] The quick rollout of COVID-19 vaccines was facilitated by advance purchase commitments.[26] It also saw the use of pooled procurement mechanisms such as COVAX and African Vaccine Acquisition Trust.[27]

The public health emergency instilled unprecedented efficiency, a proactive approach and vaccine regulators' taking huge risks. Regulators allowed clinical development before completion of prior phases. They interacted frequently with vaccine makers, which accelerated the development process. Approvals were granted based on rolling reviews[25].

mRNA: THE MAGICAL MESSENGER

One of the greatest learnings from the COVID-19 pandemic was the validation of messenger mRNA-based vaccine technology. mRNA vaccines do not deliver virus antigens to the body directly. Instead, they deliver mRNA, a molecule that instructs the host cells to produce specific viral proteins. These proteins in turn set off an immune response to fend off the virus.[28]

mRNA is like biological software. mRNA technology is amenable to the 'plug and play approach. One needs to just change the code to instruct the host cells to produce a different protein to stimulate an immune response to a different pathogen.[29]

The mRNA platform can rapidly design and produce candidate vaccines. mRNA vaccines are safe, cost-effective and scalable, produce potent immune responses and provide flexibility to modify a vaccine swiftly to take care of viral variants and emerging infections. Since mRNA vaccines are synthetic chemicals with lipid nanoparticles, their production does not have very stringent safety requirements.[30,31]

In coming years, COVID-19 mRNA vaccine-related learning will facilitate the production of mRNA vaccines against a host of pathogens.[32] Whenever a mystery pathogen emerges, scientists will quickly slot its genetic material to produce a vaccine.[33]

UNFOLDING OF A NEW GOLDEN ERA IN VACCINOLOGY

Vaccine makers are now armed with plug-and-play vaccine platforms and technologies. This has enabled rapid development, testing and production of vaccines on a large scale and in a cost-effective manner. Therefore, many new vaccines are likely to be available against existing diseases as well as new pathogens.[34,35] Scientists are also working rapidly on thermostable vaccines that do not require expensive cold-chain transport and storage. Such vaccines will be a boon for resource-constrained regions.[36]

There will also be an increase in machine-learning and computational analyses to understand the structure of a virus, identify components that contribute to an immune response, and study genetic mutation and evolution of viruses to design better vaccines.[1,37]

The world will see a transition towards broad spectrum or universal vaccines.[38,39] Substantial work has already been done on a universal influenza vaccine that will be capable of eliciting an immune response against antigenically diverse influenza viruses.[40] Duke University is developing a pan-coronavirus vaccine that will offer protection against a broad range of coronavirus infections[41,42]

Moreover, the future will see novel 'bridge vaccines, which will generate nonspecific immune responses against a variety of pathogens for which a fully effective vaccine does not exist. They will be used to decrease the rate of infection and transmission of diseases. To reduce the number of visits to get a shot, a trend to mix multiple components in a formulation is also emerging.[43]

Most of the current vaccines are administered with a hypodermic needle. Scientists are developing new and easy methods of vaccine delivery, such as nano-patches, nasal sprays, jet injectors and microneedles.[44] These will be painless, cost-effective, easy to store, simple to administer, and will reduce the amount of plastic and bio-hazardous waste.[45] We may also see more oral vaccines. The oral route activates humoral and cellular immune responses at the systemic and mucosal sites and induces a stronger and longer-lasting defence.[46]

These novel ways of administering vaccines will improve access to vaccines in rural and poor communities. They will also help in vaccinating people with trypanophobia, or fear of injections, and will thereby facilitate improved compliance.[47]

A NEW ERA OF THERAPEUTIC VACCINES

Instead of disease prevention, in the future, vaccines will also be used to treat diseases such as cancer, chronic and non-infectious diseases, and metabolic syndromes.[28] Therapeutic vaccines are used for treatment of an existing disease rather than as immunization for protection against future diseases. They utilize a patient's own immune system to fight the disease.

Future therapeutic vaccines will be based on the identification of protein markers that are unique to a disease phenotype. Personalized mRNA-encoded therapeutic proteins to cure cancer have already reached their clinical trials. In 2010, the US FDA approved the first therapeutic vaccine, Provenge, for treatment of prostate cancer. The vaccine can either be directed against the tumour itself or be designed to amplify the anti-tumour immune response.[48]

Use of vaccines to reverse vascular dysfunction of the heart, treatment of the wounds of diabetic patients, allergies, nicotine and drug addiction, and treatment of multiple sclerosis and other autoimmune diseases is being actively researched. The use of mRNA for gene therapy and to cure genetic diseases such as haemophilia and sickle-cell anaemia has also shown encouraging results. For autoimmune or allergic disorders, there will be 'negative vaccines', which will 'switch off' unwanted immune responses.[49,50,51]

Another potential use of next-generation vaccines will be to instruct cells to produce monoclonal antibodies against new unknown diseases. Therefore, if a new epidemic breaks out, blood will be taken from survivors, antibodies in their blood will be sequenced and corresponding mRNA will be produced to enable cells to produce monoclonal antibodies that will neutralize the disease-causing pathogen.[52]

ASSISTING THE UNFOLDING OF THE NEW GOLDEN AGE OF VACCINOLOGY

COVID-19 is not going to be the world's last health emergency. The world is full of pathogens. Apart from the numerous coronaviruses, there are at least 24 other virus families that can infect humans.[19] Moreover, there are existing killers for which no effective vaccine is available. Therefore, the potency of vaccines as the global arsenal to fight infectious diseases needs to be enhanced. This will require a long-term investment in basic research and knowledge accumulation of pathogens of concern.[53] It will also require physical infrastructure and clinical networks to conduct advanced research and clinical testing.[20]

The world will need nimble and ideal vaccine platforms that will allow progression from viral sequencing to clinical trials within weeks. These platforms will demonstrate a consistent immune response to different pathogens and will be suitable for large-scale production of vaccines regardless of their pathogens.[54]

Surveillance to rapidly detect and respond to new strains of pathogens and emerging zoonotic pathogens with pandemic-related potential will also be critical.[55] Pharmacovigilance of vaccines will be another critical element. All countries will need to put in place infrastructure and build their capacity for surveillance of the safety of new vaccines.[56]

Vaccines tend to be manufactured in countries with economic and technical prowess. There is an urgent need to widen the vaccine-manufacturing base in developing and low-income countries through financial support and technology transfer to facilitate equitable access to low-cost vaccines.[20,57] The affordability of vaccines is another critical factor in the fight against contagions.

As in the case of the COVID-19 vaccines, the development of future vaccines will require increased collaboration and cooperation between governments, scientists, funders, epidemiologists, developers, regulators and health authorities.[58]

Immunosuppressed individuals, such as young children, the elderly and those who are immunocompromized for medical reasons, have a limited immunogenic response to vaccines. They are very susceptible to infections and pose a formidable challenge to vaccination. Vaccines of the future need to be designed by taking care of the underlying cause of their immunosuppression.[59]

Bringing vaccines from conception to clinics swiftly will also need huge resources.[60] Also needed will be instruments to reduce business uncertainty and risk. Global legal mechanisms are needed to indemnify companies during emergencies when regulatory requirements are followed. In a promising step forward, the WHO and the World Economic Forum, with the help of the CEPI and Harvard Global Health Institute, have recently developed an insurance-based indemnification model to facilitate emergency deployment of experimental vaccines.[26] More such mechanisms will be needed to propel the growth of the vaccine industry.

COVID-19 has highlighted the challenges and consequences of misinformation and disinformation. The spread of 'infodemic' through social and digital media will encourage the mounting threat of resistance to vaccines, and significantly affect their uptake. Practices and collaborations undertaken by online platforms to counter infodemics during the COVID-19 pandemic need to be continued and enhanced while ensuring that users' rights to privacy and freedom of expression are preserved.[61]

NEW VISTAS OF GROWTH FOR INDIA'S VACCINE INDUSTRY

As vaccine-mediated control of pathogens is gaining momentum, the future of India's vaccine industry looks promising. Known for their low-cost vaccines, Indian vaccine manufacturers will play an increasingly important role in providing affordable access to effective vaccines to the world.

The Indian government's policies are friendly, especially after a complete overhaul during the COVID-19 pandemic. Speaking to me, Mr Adar Poonawalla enthusiastically confirmed, 'Today, thanks to the Modi Government, a lot of reforms have taken place, and approvals and permissions come much faster to put up new factories, and develop and launch new products.'

Indian scientists, manufacturers, regulators and government functionaries have learnt a lot in development, approval and production of COVID-19 vaccines. Apart from its traditional live attenuated and inactivated vaccines, India has also produced nucleic acid vaccines as well as viral vector vaccines to help the world fight COVID-19. India achieved the distinction of having produced the first DNA vaccine for humans that has received approval anywhere in the world.

India's vaccine-manufacturing capability is also set to get a big push through the QUAD initiative, which was aimed at accelerating the end of the COVID-19 pandemic. The QUAD partners have resolved to work collectively to expand India's capacity to manufacturing safe and effective COVID-19 vaccines. This will be used to export vaccines from India to benefit countries through the country's key multilateral initiatives, for instance, COVAX.[62]

Buoyed by the successful manufacturing of several COVID-19 vaccines, India's standing in the world vaccine market is growing. More and more foreign agencies are seeking partnerships with Indian manufacturers in the development and production of vaccines.[63]

India's Mission COVID-Suraksha is also providing financial and technical support to vaccine makers to take COVID-19 vaccines from conception to the clinic. The addition of knowledge, infrastructure and manufacturing capacity in this endeavour will definitely enhance India's standing as a global vaccine manufacturing hub. It will also equip the country to quickly roll out vaccines in the event of attacks by novel pathogens in the future.

In view of the current COVID-19 pandemic and new and emerging infectious diseases, there is tremendous scope for the Indian vaccine industry to grow in the global vaccine market for known diseases. The recent announcement of 'Immunization Agenda 2030' by the WHO, UNICEF and their development partners is good news for India. The agenda aims to bolster childhood vaccinations worldwide to cover at least 90 per cent of children. This will expand demand and aid the growth of the Indian vaccine industry.

The emerging area of therapeutic vaccines and 'bridge-vaccines' are also likely to drive the growth of the Indian vaccine industry in coming times.

Not only the global market, but the domestic Indian vaccine market also has ample potential for substantial expansion. A large number of Indian children remain unimmunized with even the most basic vaccines. Moreover, there are many new vaccines waiting for entry into India's UIP. And with the government being committed to Ayushman Bharat (healthy India), the domestic demand for vaccines is bound to increase in the months to come.

HOW CAN THE WORLD'S PHARMACIES DO BETTER?

Over the years, India's vaccine makers have built a strong credential as global producers and suppliers of life-saving vaccines. However, there are many areas where the country needs to improve to retain the nomenclature of being the 'world's pharmacy'.

According to Dr Yuvraj, Joint Secretary, Department of Pharmaceuticals, Government of India, the Indian vaccine industry is facing multiple challenges that need to be surmounted to accelerate vaccine production. 'The challenges include the lack of an adequate cold chain infrastructure, low allocation of resources by vaccine makers to research and development, limited access to state-of-the-art technologies and equipment, the evolving Intellectual Property regime, commercialization of technology and process optimization-related challenges,' he told me.

The CEO of the SII, Adar Poonawalla, while responding to my questions, sounded quite confident that the momentum gained during COVID-19 will continue in the development of vaccines for other diseases such as malaria, dengue, and so forth, and that the vaccines under development will be licensed quickly. However, according to him: 'This success can be replicated in the future if the bureaucrats and ministries continue working with the same passion in granting permission in record time as they did during the COVID-19 pandemic from 2020 to 2021.'

Quick improvement in infrastructure and our capacity for clinical trials and managing adverse events is definitely a priority. This will ensure the wide acceptance of 'Made in India' vaccines worldwide.

According to Dr Yuvraj, 'Availability of critical raw materials will continue to remain a challenge'. By their policies or laws, countries give priority to their own vaccine makers in accessing specialized materials and equipment. 'Moreover, Indian vaccine manufacturers compete with other global players for limited raw material resources', he told me.

To promote further self-sufficiency in vaccine production in the spirit of Atmanirbhar Bharat (self-reliant India), the Department of Pharmaceuticals has included vaccines under the newly launched PLI 2.0 scheme.

Another bottleneck faced by vaccine makers is that the academicians, industry and policymakers in India are used to working in vertical 'silos'. Consequently, many promising vaccine candidates, for instance, for HIV, malaria and hepatitis E, have been developed but have failed to reach the market. Therefore, for successful indigenous research, a concerted multidisciplinary and multi-stakeholder approach in the future will greatly benefit India.

One more limiting factor in vaccine research- and development-related endeavours is the availability of funding. Additional investment is urgently required in production of new vaccines and vaccine technologies.[64] The sector should also benefit from soft loans and grants from national and international agencies, and venture capitalists.

An appropriate risk-cushion mechanism for the vaccine industry is immediately needed to encourage manufacturers to take increased investment-related risks for the development of indigenous and epidemiologically suitable vaccines. In addition, the government can create an attractive ecosystem for the vaccine industry through its innovative procurement policies, long-term projections of vaccine requirements and purchase commitments.

The Indian government may also put in place GMP-compliant incubator facilities to aid start-ups in scaling up their proof-of-concept studies. Moreover, there is a need to facilitate the alignment of vaccine producers with technical and scientific institutions to further strengthen India's vaccine-manufacturing base.

One more booster for the Indian vaccine industry can come from a friendly but robust regulatory system that is in sync with international regulatory norms. A number of innovations and improvements in this arena were seen during the COVID-19 pandemic. The national regulator needs to be continuously equipped to assess new technologies, and the setting up of an accredited laboratory to support the national regulator will also be beneficial in the long run.

Vaccine manufacturers will benefit from a system for data generation and evaluation. And although VPD surveillance is being conducted by the Central Bureau of Health Intelligence and the Integrated Disease Surveillance Project, both systems have deficiencies and provide fragmented data. There is also the lack of a system to conduct post-marketing surveillance studies for new vaccines.

When I asked him about where he sees the Indian vaccine industry in 2030, Adar Poonawalla said confidently that in 2030, India will continue to lead innovation in manufacturing globally due to the country's talent pool, competitive cost base, hardworking culture and environment. 'This will always give us an edge over other countries,' he said.

With a strong and supportive government, committed academia, innovative entrepreneurs and a growing economy, it is not difficult to remove the hurdles in the way of efficient vaccine production. India's vaccine growth story is definitely poised to add many new chapters in the times to come.

REFERENCES

1. Ratanghayra N. How can we unlock new possibilities in vaccine development? [Internet]. Biopharma from Technology Networks. 2021 [cited 20 December 2021]. Available from: https://www.technologynetworks.com/biopharma/articles/how-can-we-unlock-new-possibilities-in-vaccine-development-351106
2. Walsh B. The world is not ready for the next pandemic [Internet]. TIME.com. 15 May 2017 [cited 20 December 2021]. Available from: https://time.com/magazine/us/4766607/may-15th-2017-vol-189-no-18-u-s/
3. Joi P. The next pandemic [Internet]. GAVI.org. 2021 [cited 20 December 2021]. Available from: https://www.gavi.org/vaccineswork/next-pandemic
4. Maxmen A. Has COVID taught us anything about pandemic preparedness? *Nature*. 2021:332–335.
5. De Wit E, Van Doremalen N, Falzarano D, Munster VJ. SARS and MERS: recent insights into emerging coronaviruses. *Nature Reviews Microbiology*. 2016 August;14(8):523–534.
6. Cdc.gov. Zoonotic diseases. 2021 [cited 20 December 2021]. Available from: https://www.cdc.gov/onehealth/basics/zoonotic-diseases.html#:~:text=Scientists%20estimate%20that%20more%20than,States%20and%20around%20the%20world
7. Plump A. Luck is not a strategy: The world needs to start preparing now for the next pandemic [Internet]. STAT. 2021 [cited 20 December 2021]. Available from: https://www.statnews.com/2021/05/18/luck-is-not-a-strategy-the-world-needs-to-start-preparing-now-for-the-next-pandemic/

8. Lauring AS, Andino R. Quasispecies theory and the behavior of RNA viruses. *PLoS Pathogens*. 2010 July 22;6(7):e1001005.
9. Lipkin WI, Firth C. Viral surveillance and discovery. *Current Opinion in Virology*. 2013 April 1;3(2):199–204.
10. Settele J, Díaz S, Brondizio E, Daszak P. COVID-19 stimulus measures must save lives, protect livelihoods, and safeguard nature to reduce the risk of future pandemics. *IBPES Expert Guest Article*. 2020 April 27;27.
11. Crooke SN, Ovsyannikova IG, Poland GA, Kennedy RB. Immunosenescence and human vaccine immune responses. *Immunity & Ageing*. 2019 December;16(1):1–6.
12. Akha AA. Aging and the immune system: An overview. *Journal of Immunological Methods*. 2018 December 1;463:21–6.
13. Cai Z, Yang Y, Zhang J. Obesity is associated with severe disease and mortality in patients with Coronavirus disease 2019 (COVID-19): A meta-analysis. *BMC Public Health*. 2021 December 1;(1):1–4.
14. Buchy P, Buisson Y, Cintra O, Dwyer DE, Nissen M, de Lejarazu RO, Petersen E. Covid-19 pandemic: Lessons learned from more than a century of pandemics and current vaccine development for pandemic control. *International Journal of Infectious Diseases*. 2021 November 1;112:300–17.
15. Air transport, passengers carried [Internet]. Data.worldbank.org. 2021 [cited 20 December 2021]. Available from: https://data.worldbank.org/indicator/IS.AIR.PSGR
16. World's population increasingly urban with more than half living in urban areas [Internet]. United Nations Department of Economic and Social Affairs. 2021 [cited 20 December 2021]. Available from: https://www.un.org/en/development/desa/news/population/world-urbanization-prospects-2014.html
17. Climate change [Internet]. WHO.int. 2021 [cited 20 December 2021]. Available from: https://www.who.int/health-topics/climate-change#tab=tab_1
18. Bedford J, Farrar J, Ihekweazu C, Kang G, Koopmans M, Nkengasong J. A new twenty-first century science for effective epidemic response. *Nature*. 2019 November;575(7781):130–136.
19. Ball P. The lightning-fast quest for COVID vaccines and what it means for other diseases. *Nature*. 2021 January 7;589:16–18.
20. Bok K, Sitar S, Graham BS, Mascola JR. Accelerated COVID-19 vaccine development: Milestones, lessons and prospects. *Immunity*. 2021 August 10;54(8):1636–1651.
21. Malone B, Simovski B, Moliné C, Cheng J, Gheorghe M, Fontenelle H, et al. Artificial intelligence predicts the immunogenic landscape of SARS-CoV-2 leading to universal blueprints for vaccine designs. *Scientific Reports*. 2020 December 23;10(1):1–4.
22. Vasan S, Pitisuttithum P. Vaccine development lessons between HIV and COVID-19. *The Lancet Infectious Diseases*. 2021 June 1;21(6):759–761.

23. Wu F, Zhao S, Yu B, Chen YM, Wang W, Song ZG, et al. A new coronavirus associated with human respiratory disease in China. *Nature.* 2020 March;579(7798):265–269.
24. Chakraborty C, Sharma AR, Bhattacharya M, Lee SS. Lessons learned from cutting-edge immunoinformatics on next-generation COVID-19 vaccine research. *International Journal of Peptide Research and Therapeutics.* 2021 December;27(4):2303–2311.
25. Insights on Life Sciences [Internet]. www.mckinsey.com. 2021 [cited 20 December 2021]. Available from: https://www.mckinsey.com/industries/life-sciences/our-insights
26. Billington J, Deschamps I, Erck SC, Gerberding JL, Hanon E, Ivol S. Developing vaccines for SARS-CoV-2 and future epidemics and pandemics: Applying lessons from past outbreaks. *Health Security.* 2020 June 1;18(3):241–249.
27. Uribe J, Basu P, Lindelow M. Preparing for the next pandemic: What will it take? [Internet]. World Bank Blogs. 2021 [cited 20 December 2021]. Available from: https://blogs.worldbank.org/voices/preparing-next-pandemic-what-will-it-take
28. Mu Z, Haynes BF, Cain DW. HIV mRNA vaccines—Progress and future paths. *Vaccines.* 2021 February;9(2):134.
29. Karikó K. In vitro-transcribed mRNA therapeutics: Out of the shadows and into the spotlight. *Mol Ther.* 2019;27(4):691–692.
30. Dolgin E. How COVID unlocked the power of RNA vaccines. *Nature.* 2021;589(7841):189–191.
31. Maruggi G, Zhang C, Li J, Ulmer JB, Yu D. mRNA as a transformative technology for vaccine development to control infectious diseases. *Mol Ther.* 2019 April 10;27:757–772.
32. Wang Y, Zhang Z, Luo J, Han X, Wei Y, Wei X. mRNA vaccine: A potential therapeutic strategy. *Molecular Cancer.* 2021 December;20(1):1–23.
33. Yong E. How science beat the virus [Internet]. *The Atlantic.* 2021 [cited 20 December 2021]. Available from: https://www.theatlantic.com/magazine/archive/2021/01/science-covid-19-manhattan-project/617262/
34. van Riel D, de Wit E. Next-generation vaccine platforms for COVID-19. *Nature Materials.* 2020 August;19(8):810–812.
35. Karikó K, Whitehead K, van der Meel R. What does the success of mRNA vaccines tell us about the future of biological therapeutics? *Cell Systems.* 2021 August 18;12(8):757.
36. Isanaka S, Guindo O, Langendorf C, Matar Seck A, Plikaytis BD, Sayinzoga-Makombe N, et al. Efficacy of a low-cost, heat-stable oral rotavirus vaccine in Niger. *New England Journal of Medicine.* 2017 March 23;376(12):1121–1130.
37. Yang Z, Bogdan P, Nazarian S. An in silico deep learning approach to multi-epitope vaccine design: a SARS-CoV-2 case study. *Scientific Reports.* 2021 February 5;11(1):1–21.

38. Marston HD, Paules CI, Fauci AS. The critical role of biomedical research in pandemic preparedness. Jama. 2017 November 14;318(18):1757–1758.
39. Cassone A, Rappuoli R. Universal vaccines: Shifting to one for many. *MBio.* 2010 May 18;1(1):e00042–10.
40. Ostrowsky J, Arpey M, Moore K, Osterholm M, Friede M, Gordon J, et al. Tracking progress in universal influenza vaccine development. *Current Opinion in Virology.* 2020 February 1;40:28–36.
41. Researchers discuss new vaccine that could prevent future pandemics [Internet]. Today.duke.edu. 2021 [cited 20 December 2021]. Available from: https://today.duke.edu/2021/05/researchers-discuss-new-vaccine-could-prevent-future-pandemics
42. Buchy P, Buisson Y, Cintra O, Dwyer DE, Nissen M, de Lejarazu RO et al. Covid-19 pandemic: Lessons learned from more than a century of pandemics and current vaccine development for pandemic control. *International Journal of Infectious Diseases.* 2021 November 1;112:300–317.
43. The global future of vaccines [Internet]. *The Guardian.* 2021 [cited 20 December 2021]. Available from: https://www.theguardian.com/vax-facts/2021/oct/13/vaccines-future-coronavirus-pandemics
44. Gutierrez A. Changing the route of vaccine administration [Internet]. *Biopharma from Technology Networks.* 2021 [cited 20 December 2021]. Available from: https://www.technologynetworks.com/biopharma/articles/changing-up-the-route-of-vaccine-administration-349321
45. Ramirez JE, Sharpe LA, Peppas NA. Current state and challenges in developing oral vaccines. *Advanced Drug Delivery Reviews.* 2017 May 15;114:116–131.
46. Patel A, Ramani R. A review on current status and future prospectus of oral vaccines. Available from: https://www.journalajmah.com/index.php/AJMAH/article/view/30342
47. Dong C, Wang Y, Gonzalez GX, Ma Y, Song Y, Wang S, et al. Intranasal vaccination with influenza HA/GO-PEI nanoparticles provides immune protection against homo-and heterologous strains. *Proceedings of the National Academy of Sciences.* 2021 May 11;118(19).
48. Shahnazari M, Samadi P, Pourjafar M, Jalali A. Therapeutic vaccines for colorectal cancer: the progress and future prospect. *International Immunopharmacology.* 2020 November 1;88:106944.
49. Nossal GJ. Vaccines of the future. *Vaccine.* 2011 December 30;29:D111–115.
50. What does the future hold for vaccination? Australian Academy of Science [Internet]. Science.org.au. 2021 [cited 20 December 2021]. Available from: https://www.science.org.au/education/immunisation-climate-change-genetic-modification/science-immunisation/5-what-does-future
51. Dorofeeva Y, Shilovskiy I, Tulaeva I, Focke-Tejkl M, Flicker S, Kudlay D, et al. Past, present, and future of allergen immunotherapy vaccines. *Allergy.* 2021 January;76(1):131–149.

52. Ruffell D. The future in an RNA molecule: From mRNA vaccines to therapeutics. An interview with Drew Weissman. *FEBS Letters*. 2021 September;595(18): 2305–2309.
53. Graham BS, Sullivan NJ. Emerging viral diseases from a vaccinology perspective: Preparing for the next pandemic. *Nature Immunology*. 2018 January;19(1):20–28.
54. Lurie N, Saville M, Hatchett R, Halton J. Developing Covid-19 vaccines at pandemic speed. *New England Journal of Medicine*. 2020 May 21;382(21):1969–1973.
55. Carlson CJ. From predict to prevention, one pandemic later. *The Lancet Microbe*. 2020 May 1;1(1):e6–7.
56. World Health Organization. Covid-19 vaccines: Safety surveillance manual. 2020. Available from: https://apps.who.int/iris/handle/10665/338400
57. Vu MN, Kelly HG, Kent SJ, Wheatley AK. Current and future nanoparticle vaccines for Covid-19. *EBioMedicine*. 2021 December 1;74:103699.
58. Excler JL, Saville M, Berkley S, Kim JH. Vaccine development for emerging infectious diseases. *Nature Medicine*. 2021 April;27(4):591–600.
59. Domínguez-Andrés J, van Crevel R, Divangahi M, Netea MG. Designing the next generation of vaccines: Relevance for future pandemics. *MBio*. 2020 December 22;11(6):e02616–2620.
60. Kis Z, Shattock R, Shah N, Kontoravdi C. Emerging technologies for low-cost, rapid vaccine manufacture. *Biotechnology Journal*. 2019 January;14(1):1800376.
61. Combatting COVID-19 disinformation on online platforms [Internet]. OECD. 2021 [cited 20 December 2021]. Available from: https://www.oecd.org/coronavirus/policy-responses/combatting-covid-19-disinformation-on-online-platforms-d854ec48/
62. Fact sheet: Quad summit [Internet]. The White House. 2021 [cited 20 December 2021]. Available from: https://www.whitehouse.gov/briefing-room/statements-releases/2021/03/12/fact-sheet-quad-summit/
63. Does the future look bright for India´s vaccine industry? [Internet]. https://www.farmantra.com/. 2021 [cited 20 December 2021]. Available from: https://www.farmantra.com/blog/does-the-future-look-bright-for-indias-vaccine-industry/
64. Pardi N, Hogan MJ, Porter FW, Weissman D. mRNA vaccines—a new era in vaccinology. *Nature Reviews Drug Discovery*. April 2018. 17(4):261–279.

Glossary

Adjuvant: An ingredient used in some vaccines that helps to create a stronge immune response in people receiving the vaccine

Anaphylaxis : An acute, potentially life-threatening hypersensitivity reaction

Antigen: A toxin or other foreign substance that induces an immune response in the body, especially the production of antibodies (*Oxford Dictionary*)

Antiserum (plural antisera): Blood serum that contains antibodies against an infective agent (such as a bacteria or virus) or toxic substance (such as snake venom) and may be used to prevent or treat infection or poisoning (*Merriam-Webster*)

Bioinformatics: Collection, classification, storage and analysis of biochemical and biological information using computers, especially as applied to molecular genetics and genomics (*Merriam-Webster*)

Efficacy: Efficacy of a vaccine is the proportionate reduction in disease among a vaccinated group

Emergency use authorization: An authorization whereby certain unapproved medical products or unapproved uses of approved medical products may be used in an emergency to diagnose, treat or prevent serious or life-threatening diseases or conditions caused by biologic, chemical or nuclear agents when there are no adequate approved and available alternatives (lawinsider.com)

Epidemic: An increase, often sudden, in the number of cases of a disease above what is normally expected in the population in an area (Centers for Disease Control and Prevention)

Genome: The complete set of genetic information in an organism, which provides all of the information the organism requires to function

Genomics: A branch of biotechnology concerned with applying the techniques of genetics and molecular biology to the genetic mapping and DNA sequencing of sets of genes or the complete genomes of selected organisms, with organization of the results in databases and applications of the data (*Merriam-Webster*)

Immune system: A complex network of cells, tissues, organs and substances they make that helps the body fight infections and other diseases (cancer.gov)

Immunization: A process by which a person is protected against a disease through vaccination, the term being often used interchangeably with vaccination or inoculation (Centers for Disease Control and Prevention)

Immunoinformatics: The science that studies immunogenetics and immunology data by using a bioinformatics and computational approach (springer.com)

Immunomics: The study of all the antigens present in particular biological specimens and approaches that can be used to identify these or use them as potential targets for treatment (*Medical Dictionary*)

Immunosenescence : Alteration of immune functions due to ageing (sciencedirect.com)

Immunosuppression : Suppression of the body's immune system and its ability to fight infections and other diseases (cancer.gov)

Index case: The patient in an outbreak who is first noticed by the health authorities and who makes them aware that an outbreak may be emerging (Lancet)

Infodemic : Too much information including false or misleading data in digital and physical environments during a disease outbreak, which causes confusion and risk-taking behaviour that can harm health and also lead to mistrust in health authorities and undermine the public health response (WHO)

Inoculation: A broad term that means to implant a virus, as is done in vaccines, or even to implant a toxic or harmful microorganism into something as a part of scientific research (dictionary.com)

Morbidity: The state of having a specific illness or condition (healthline.com)

Mutation: A permanent change or a structural alteration in the DNA or RNA (medicine.net)

Pandemic: An epidemic occurring worldwide or over a very wide area, crossing international boundaries and usually affecting a large number of people (*A Dictionary of Epidemiology*)

Pharmacovigilance: The science and activities relating to the detection, assessment, understanding and prevention of adverse effects or any other medicine- or vaccine-related problem (WHO)

Proteomics: A branch of biotechnology concerned with applying the techniques of molecular biology, biochemistry and genetics to analyse the structure, function and interactions of the proteins produced by the genes of a particular cell, tissue or organism, organizing the information as well as the applications of the data in databases (*Merriam-Webster*)

Public health: The approach to medicine that is concerned with the health of the community as a whole (medicinenet.com)

Public Health Emergency of International Concern: An extraordinary event that is determined to constitute a public health risk to other states through the international spread of a disease, which potentially requires a coordinated international response (WHO)

Serotype: Groups within a single species of microorganisms such as bacteria or viruses, which share distinctive surface structures (Centers for Disease Control and Prevention)

Serum: The clear liquid that can be separated from clotted blood (differing from plasma), the liquid portion of normal unclotted blood containing the red and white cells and platelets, the clot making the difference between serum and plasma (medicinenet.com)

Strain: A genetic variant or subtype of a microorganism, for instance, a virus, bacterium or fungus

Vaccination: The act of introducing a vaccine into a body to protect it from a specific disease (Centers for Disease Control and Prevention)

Vaccine: A preparation that is used to stimulate the body's immune response against diseases; usually administered through needle injections, but some being administered by mouth or sprayed into the nose (Centers for Disease Control and Prevention)

Vaccinology: The science of vaccines (nature.com)

Variant: A viral genome (genetic code) that may contain one or more mutations (Centers for Disease Control and Prevention)

Variant of concern: A variant for which there is evidence of an increase in its transmissibility, which is a severe disease (for instance, increased hospitalization or death), there is a significant reduction in neutralization by antibodies generated by previous infection or vaccination, the reduced effectiveness of treatments or vaccines, or diagnostic detection failures (Centers for Disease Control and Prevention)

Variant of interest: A variant with specific genetic markers that have been associated with changes in receptor binding, reduced neutralization by antibodies generated by previous infection or vaccination, the reduced efficacy of treatments, the potential diagnostic impact, a predicted increase in transmissibility or serious disease (Centers for Disease Control and Prevention)

Variolation: The old practice of inoculating a person with the virus of smallpox to produce immunity to the disease (medicinenet.com)

Virus: An infective agent that typically consists of a nucleic acid molecule in a protein coat, which is too small to be seen by light microscopy and is able to only multiply within the living cells of a host (Lexico.com)

About the Author

Sajjan Yadav is a researcher and a bureaucrat. He is an officer of the Indian Administrative Service and is currently Additional Secretary in the Department of Expenditure, Ministry of Finance, Government of India.

He has a rich and diverse experience of 27 years in policy formulation and implementation, as well as in senior leadership positions in the Government of India and state governments. In the federal government, besides the Ministry of Finance, he has worked in the Ministry of Health and Family Welfare, Ministry of Women & Child Development, Ministry of Heavy Industry and Public Enterprises, and Ministry of Corporate Affairs

He has served the government in sectors including finance, health, nutrition, water, sanitation, food, public distribution, urban development, municipal administration, information and publicity, art, culture, tourism and commercial taxes. Important assignments handled by him in the past include tenures as Mission Director of the National Nutrition Mission (POSHAN Abhiyan), Director of the National Rural Health Mission, Commissioner of Food & Supplies in Delhi, CEO Delhi Jal Board, Commissioner VAT and Commissioner of the East Delhi Municipal Corporation.

He earned his Doctorate in Public Health from the prestigious London School of Hygiene and Tropical Medicine (LSHTM). His research was published in leading medical peer-reviewed journals, magazines and newspapers. These include *BMC Public Health*, *Indian Journal of Medical Research*, *Indian Journal of Occupational and Environmental Medicine*, *International Journal of Medicine and Public Health*, *Journal of Critical Reviews*, *LSHTM Research Online*, *Global*

Health Action, *Yojana*, *The Economic Times*, *DNA*, *Millennium Post* and *The Pioneer*.

He has been conferred many awards for exceptional work in public service, including the National e-Governance Award 2017–2018 and the President of India's medal for outstanding work in Census operations.